Evaluation and Management of High-Risk Pregnancies:

Emerging Research and Opportunities

Sapna Nanda
Panjab University, India

A volume in the Advances in Medical Diagnosis, Treatment, and Care (AMDTC) Book Series

IGI Global
PUBLISHER of TIMELY KNOWLEDGE

Published in the United States of America by
IGI Global
Medical Information Science Reference (an imprint of IGI Global)
701 E. Chocolate Avenue
Hershey PA, USA 17033
Tel: 717-533-8845
Fax: 717-533-8661
E-mail: cust@igi-global.com
Web site: http://www.igi-global.com

Library of Congress Cataloging-in-Publication Data

Names: Nanda, Sapna, 1964- author.
Title: Evaluation and management of high-risk pregnancies : emerging research and opportunities / by Sapna Nanda.
Description: Hershey, PA : Medical Information Science Reference, [2020] | Includes bibliographical references and index. | Summary: "This book explores the diagnosis, treatment, and management of high-risk pregnancies"-- Provided by publisher.
Identifiers: LCCN 2019059986 (print) | LCCN 2019059987 (ebook) | ISBN 9781799843573 (hardcover) | ISBN 9781799843580 (ebook)
Subjects: MESH: Pregnancy, High-Risk | Pregnancy Complications--diagnosis | Pregnancy Complications--therapy | Maternal Death--prevention & control
Classification: LCC RG571 (print) | LCC RG571 (ebook) | NLM WQ 240 | DDC 618.3--dc23
LC record available at https://lccn.loc.gov/2019059986
LC ebook record available at https://lccn.loc.gov/2019059987

This book is published in the IGI Global book series Advances in Medical Diagnosis, Treatment, and Care (AMDTC) (ISSN: 2475-6628; eISSN: 2475-6636)

British Cataloguing in Publication Data
A Cataloguing in Publication record for this book is available from the British Library.

For electronic access to this publication, please contact: eresources@igi-global.com.

Advances in Medical Diagnosis, Treatment, and Care (AMDTC) Book Series

ISSN:2475-6628
EISSN:2475-6636

MISSION

Advancements in medicine have prolonged the life expectancy of individuals all over the world. Once life-threatening conditions have become significantly easier to treat and even cure in many cases. Continued research in the medical field will further improve the quality of life, longevity, and wellbeing of individuals.

The **Advances in Medical Diagnosis, Treatment, and Care (AMDTC)** book series seeks to highlight publications on innovative treatment methodologies, diagnosis tools and techniques, and best practices for patient care. Comprised of comprehensive resources aimed to assist professionals in the medical field apply the latest innovations in the identification and management of medical conditions as well as patient care and interaction, the books within the AMDTC series are relevant to the research and practical needs of medical practitioners, researchers, students, and hospital administrators.

COVERAGE

- Internal Medicine
- Diagnostic Medicine
- Disease Management
- Patient Interaction
- Patient-Centered Care
- Emergency Medicine
- Critical Care
- Alternative Medicine
- Medical Testing
- Medical Procedures

IGI Global is currently accepting manuscripts for publication within this series. To submit a proposal for a volume in this series, please contact our Acquisition Editors at Acquisitions@igi-global.com or visit: http://www.igi-global.com/publish/.

The Advances in Medical Diagnosis, Treatment, and Care (AMDTC) Book Series (ISSN 2475-6628) is published by IGI Global, 701 E. Chocolate Avenue, Hershey, PA 17033-1240, USA, www.igi-global.com. This series is composed of titles available for purchase individually; each title is edited to be contextually exclusive from any other title within the series. For pricing and ordering information please visit http://www.igi-global.com/book-series/advances-medical-diagnosis-treatment-care/129618. Postmaster: Send all address changes to above address.

Titles in this Series

For a list of additional titles in this series, please visit:
https://www.igi-global.com/book-series/advances-medical-diagnosis-treatment-care/129618

Noninvasive Ventilation Technologies and Healthcare for Geriatric Patients
César Fonseca (Universidade de Évora, Portugal) Manuel José Lopes (Universidade de Évora, Portugal) David Mendes (Universidade de Évora, Portugal) Jose Garcia-Alonso (University of Extremadura, Spain) and Felismina Mendes (Universidade de Évora, ortugal)
Medical Information Science Reference • © 2020 • 252pp • H/C (ISBN: 9781799835318) • US $245.00

Diagnostic and Treatment Methods for Ulcerative Colitis and Colitis-Associaed Cancer
Ashok Kumar Pandurangan (B.S. Abdur Rahman Crescent Institute of Science and Technology, India)
Medical Information Science Reference • © 2020 • 300pp • H/C (ISBN: 9781799835806) • US $295.00

Biopsychosocial Perspectives and Practices for Addressing Communicable and Non-Communicable Diseases
Simon George Taukeni (University of Namibia, Namibia)
Medical Information Science Reference • © 2020 • 368pp • H/C (ISBN: 9781799821397) • US $265.00

Role of Nutrition in Providing Pro-/Anti-Inflammatory Balance Emerging Research and Opportunities
Uğur Günşen (Bandırma Onyedi Eylül University, Turkey) and Ramazan Mert Atan (Bandırma Onyedi Eylül University, Turkey)
Medical Information Science Reference • © 2020 • 214pp • H/C (ISBN: 9781799835943) • US $235.00

Handbook of Research on Prenatal, Postnatal, and Early Childhood Development
Neriman Aral (Ankara University, Turkey)
Medical Information Science Reference • © 2020 • 470pp • H/C (ISBN: 9781799829522) • US $365.00

IGI Global
PUBLISHER of TIMELY KNOWLEDGE

701 East Chocolate Avenue, Hershey, PA 17033, USA
Tel: 717-533-8845 x100 • Fax: 717-533-8661
E-Mail: cust@igi-global.com • www.igi-global.com

Table of Contents

Foreword

Pregnancy, a woman's privilege, is the means for survival of the human species. Women have a right to safe motherhood, when they risk their lives and health in order to give birth to a new life. Pregnancy should not compete for vital resources with the pathological conditions. Pregnancy is, thus, very special.

However, in some parts of the world, women continue to face difficult circumstances surrounding pregnancy and childbirth. Just like many other women, the pregnant women have the same hopes and fears about having a child. Unfortunately, their fears are well-founded. But, so are their hopes.

In the past, pregnancy and childbirth were more dangerous. But, today, it's so much safer to have a baby. If one gets regular prenatal care, eats well, makes good lifestyle choices and have an institutional delivery or a skilled health practitioner at the time of delivery, the chances of having a healthy pregnancy and child birth are excellent.

In countries with a good economy, modern technology and access to healthcare, the chances of dying during pregnancy, during childbirth or in the days or weeks after delivery are very low. In developed countries such as the United States, the United Kingdom and Canada, most women have healthy pregnancies and child births. Of course, there is still a small risk of maternal mortality and morbidity, even in developed countries. In developed countries, dying during childbirth or because of pregnancy is very rare, even if the pregnancy is high-risk.

According to the Centers for Disease Control (CDC), approximately 700 women a year lose their lives from complications having to do with pregnancy in the United States (Centers for Disease Control and Prevention, 2019). Health officials report the rate of maternal mortality as to how many women die for every 1,00, 000 live births. There are around 4 million births in the United States each year and during the year 2015; there were approximately 17 maternal deaths for every 100,000 live births (Centers for Disease Control and Prevention, 2019). In the United States, the chances of dying because of pregnancy are at most approximately 1 in 3500.

Other developed countries have similar and even lower maternal mortality rates when compared to the United States. However, that is not the case everywhere. Throughout the world, over 3, 00,000 women die each year from the complications that arise during pregnancy and childbirth whereas about 700 women die each year in the United States, the World Health Organization (WHO) reports that approximately 830 women die each day worldwide (World Health Organization, 2019).

Most of these women worldwide (almost 99 percent) live in poor and impoverished conditions in the developing countries. In some countries, the odds of dying because of pregnancy are as high as 1 death among 15 women. And, the sad fact is that many of these deaths are preventable (World Health Organization, 2019).

This alarming rate of maternal mortality could be attributed to the fact that a substantial proportion of teen births are intended in developing countries where many women still marry early (Kothari et al, 2012). However, even intended pregnancies among young women in low resource settings are of policy and public health relevance because of the high risks associated with them. The risk of death associated with pregnancy is about a third higher among 15 to 19 year olds than among 20 to 24 year olds (Nove et al, 2012). It appears that young adolescents are more likely to experience obstructed labor, fistula and premature delivery and to give birth to low birth weight babies than older women (UNFPA, 2013).

Adolescents are, thus, more seriously affected by complications of pregnancy than older women (World Health Organization, 2014). The physically devastating potential consequences of unsafe abortions include cervical tearing, perforated uterus and bowel, hemorrhage, chronic pelvic infection and abscesses, infertility, endotoxic shock, renal failure and death. The long-term sequelae include ectopic pregnancy, chronic pelvic pain, and infertility (Ibrahim and Onwudiegwu, 2012). Potential discrimination and rejection by family or community members, psychosocial stress, forced marriage and violence often impact these young women (World Health Organization, 2007).

Irrespective of the magnitude of the increased risk of maternal mortality and morbidity for young adolescents, many overwhelming reasons exist for young adolescent women to avoid early childbearing, including the widespread adverse social, educational and economic consequences for young adolescent mothers.

In such a scenario, many maternal and child health organizations such as WHO, USAID, UNICEF, UNFPA and many others are bringing awareness to this issue. These organizations are developing maternal and child health programs to help fight maternal mortality and morbidity so as to make the future better for all women. For reproductive health services to be woman-friendly, they have to recognize and respond to the continuum of reproductive health care needs, they have to see the woman behind the mother, they have to see women as ends and not means and they have to tailor their services according to the women's needs and perceptions.

World Health Organization report (2005) reviews the three most important ways in which the outcomes of pregnancies can be improved which include providing good antenatal care, finding appropriate ways of preventing and dealing with the consequences of unwanted pregnancies, and improving the way society looks after pregnant women.

This manuscript is an attempt to focus on the emerging research and opportunities that provide the vital tools which women need to help them plan their pregnancy, negotiate the changes they will experience and develop a safe and appropriate birth plan. It will also provide the much needed information for the care givers and health professionals to ensure the necessary support for the successful outcome of their pregnancies. Additionally, it will help the policy makers and planners of various maternal and child health programmes to strategize the interventions for safe and healthy motherhood and the institutional deliveries that will ensure the baby the best possible start in life.

Neelam Aggarwal
PGIMER, Chandigarh, India

REFERENCES

Centers for Disease Control and Prevention. (2019a). *Pregnancy-Related Deaths*. Author.

Centers for Disease Control and Prevention. (2019b). *Pregnancy mortality Surveillance System*. Author.

Ibrahim, I. A., & Onwudiegwu, U. (2012). Socio-demographic determinants of complicated unsafe abortions in a semi-urban Nigerian town: A four-year review. *The West Indian Medical Journal*, *61*(2), 163–167. PMID:23155964

Kothari, M. T., Wang, S., & Head, S. (2012). *Trends in adolescent reproductive and sexual behaviors. DHS Comparative Reports No. 29*. ICF International.

Nove, A., Matthews, Z. & Neal, S. (2012). Maternal mortality in adolescents compared with women of other ages: Evidence from 144 countries. *The Lancet Global Health*, *2*, e155-e64.

UNFPA. (2013). *Motherhood in childhood: Facing the challenge of adolescent pregnancy: The State of World Population 2013*. United Nations Population Fund.

World Health Organization. (2007). *Adolescent pregnancy: unmet needs and undone deeds: A review of the literature and programmes*. WHO.

World Health Organization. (2014). *Adolescent pregnancy. Fact sheet No. 364*. https://www.who.int/mediacentre/factsheets/fs364/en/

World Health Organization. (2019). *Maternal Mortality*. WHO.

World Health Report. (2005). *Make Every Woman and Child Count*. Author.

Preface

The gestation period is a period of rapid growth and development. Growth of the foetus and other developments that take place to facilitate its maintenance throughout pregnancy and delivery of the child involves an increase in the nutritional and health needs of the pregnant women.

The needs of pregnant women had been traditionally addressed within the concept of Maternal and Child Health (MCH). The needs of a woman were submerged in the needs of a mother. Maternal and Child Health programs and services have been playing and still continue to play an important role in promotive, preventive and curative health care of mothers and children.

All the Maternal and Child Health (MCH) care services tend to focus primarily on the healthy child as the successful outcome of pregnancy. While mothers care very much for this successful outcome because of the investment they make in the process of reproduction, this focus resulted in less emphasis being put on caring for the health risks to which mothers themselves are subjected to during pregnancy and childbirth and on putting in place the essential obstetric functions and facilities to overcome them. As a result, the tragedy of maternal mortality and morbidity in developing countries has now reached the dimension that can no longer be ignored.

The tragedy of maternal mortality and morbidity in developing countries is not just a health problem; it should be recognized as a human rights issue. The theme for World Health Day in the year 1998 was "Pregnancy is Special; Let's make it safe". When the World Health Assembly adopted this theme, it was setting a principle in health policy. Pregnancy is not a disease. Pregnancy is special (WHO, 1998).

However, the concept of Maternal and Child Health (MCH) focuses a special attention on women only when and if they are reproducing so as to ensure that they produce healthy children but often neglects their other reproduction-related health needs. Women's reproduction-related health needs are not only limited to the reproductive years of their lives. The girl child, the adolescent girl, the mature adult and older woman have their stage-specific health and other needs which relate either to their past or future reproductive functions.

With women considered as means and not as ends, important health and other needs of women in the reproductive functions have been left unmet. Infertility in itself may not be a serious health hazard as far as physical health of women is concerned but it can be a major cause of mental, psychological and social ill-health. It is, thus, not just fair that society provides care to the reproducing women but neglects the suffering of those who are unable to conceive.

The societal attitude of looking at women as means and not as ends is even more pervasive. Services usually offered to women often have something of a very poor quality. Even the proponents of education of girl state the advantages of education that such education will ensure the survival and health of the children and the impact it will have on reducing the birth rate. Nutrition of pregnant and lactating women is justified because of the needs of the foetus and the breastfed infant. Even with the tragedy of maternal mortality, a justification put forward for investment in keeping mothers alive is that their survival is critical for the survival of their children.

Although during infancy and early childhood, girls and boys suffer from broadly similar health problems, striking sex differentials emerge during adulthood. Women suffer disproportionately due to their reproductive role. Although the burden of reproductive ill-health is almost entirely confined to the developing regions, it is so great that even worldwide, reproductive conditions make up three out of the ten leading causes of disease burden in women, aged between 15 and 44 years. In the developing countries, five out of the ten leading causes of DALY's (Disability-Adjusted Life Years) are related to reproductive ill-health, including the consequences of unsafe abortions and infections. Almost all of this loss of healthy life is avoidable (Murray and Lopez, 1996).

In a joint major exercise of the World Health Organization and the World Bank, quantitative assessments were made of the global burden of different diseases and the results were expressed in the terms of disability-adjusted life years (DALY's) lost as a result of the disease (World Bank, 1993).

The burden of a disease is primarily a function of its prevalence and its seriousness to the individual concerned. However, in the case of reproductive health, the impact is not only limited to the individual directly concerned but also to the future generations. The health of the child will have an impact on the health of the adult. Investment in reproductive health of women is, thus, an investment in the future generations.

The concept of "reproductive health" has recently emerged in response to the fragmentation of the existing health services and their orientation. The broader concept of "reproductive health" offers a comprehensive and integrated approach to the health needs related to reproduction. It puts women at the center of the process, as subjects and not as objects, as ends and not as means. It recognizes respects and responds to the reproductive health needs of the woman behind the mother.

Adolescent sexual and reproductive health (ASRH) has been overlooked historically despite the high risks that countries face for its neglect. Some of the challenges faced by adolescents across the world include early pregnancy and parenthood, difficulties accessing contraception and safe abortion and high rates of HIV and sexually transmitted infections. Various political, economic, and socio-cultural factors restrict the delivery of information and services; healthcare workers often act as a barrier to care by failing to provide young people with supportive, non-judgmental, youth-appropriate services (Morris and Rushwan, 2015).

Country-specific estimates of pregnancy, childbirth and abortion levels among adolescents can motivate policy and programmatic responses to teenage pregnancies and help monitor progress toward reducing their incidence. Countries with low levels of adolescent pregnancy might serve as references or models for efforts to reduce levels elsewhere. Even where incidence is low, data on teenage pregnancies can highlight the remaining unmet needs for information and services to help adolescents prevent unintended pregnancies (Sedgh et al., 2015).

With all the benefits to the quality of life of women, family planning programs have left women with some genuine concerns as well as unmet needs (Fathalla, 1994). Women have more at stake in fertility control than anyone else. Contraceptives are meant to be used by women to empower themselves by maximizing their choices and controlling their fertility, their sexuality, their reproductive health needs and thus their overall lives.

Moreover, sexual relationships expose women to the risk of unwanted pregnancies. These unwanted pregnancies expose many women to another serious or more serious risk, that of sexually-transmitted infections, including HIV infection. Family planning programs, with an exclusive demographic focus, do not focus on the issue of this important health need of women.

Family planning programs, however, can be used and have been used by the government and other agencies to control rather than to empower women. The family planning movement in many countries has been largely demographic driven. As far as planners and policymakers are concerned, women were often treated as objects and not as subjects. Some governments were even short-sighted, not to see that when women are given a real choice and the information and means to implement their choice, they will make the most rational decision for themselves, for their families, for their communities, for their nations and ultimately for the world at large.

Inability of most of the women and couples in the developing countries so as to regulate and control their fertility because of lack of information and inadequacy of services is not only affecting the health of the people immediately concerned and their families but has implications for their communities and their nations, for global stability and for the balance between population and natural resources and between the human species and the environment.

A strong case can, thus, be made for the integration of all reproductive health care services at the level of planning and policy making, management and administration so as to ensure that all these reproductive health needs of women receive an immediate attention and a relatively adequate allocation of resources. Reproductive health care, thus, should be an integrated package. There are, however, two levels for integration. Services can be integrated at the level of planning and policy making, management and administration and/or at the level of service delivery.

At the level of service delivery, it must be ensured that the approach should be pragmatic. Services should be integrated only if the integration of services makes their delivery more cost-effective. Different situations in countries should be evaluated and assessed on their own, taking into consideration some basic principles. Service delivery should be more cost-effective either through optimum utilization of services, resulting in an increase of output or cost savings resulting in a decrease of inputs.

Better utilization of services can result only when integration of services makes services more convenient and accessible to the beneficiaries. It can also happen when the demand on one service can increase or create a demand for the other, e.g. the demand for child care may increase the demand for family planning and so on.

Cost savings can be done when fixed costs are shared between different services. This can happen if the same infra-structure can be used for the different services to be integrated, if the services can be provided by the same service providers and if enough excess capacity is available to meet the demands of the new service to be added.

However, integration of services should be distinguished from "bundling" of services. The verb "bundle "(a common computer software jargon) is defined as "tie in, make up into, a bundle; throw confusedly in to any receptacle". When services are simply combined or joined together in one way or another, this is, not necessarily, integration. In such cases, it may be more appropriately labeled as bundling. When services are combined or joined together as a strategy to provide a more complete package for services needed, this is integration.

The need for comprehensive health care should not translate to an all or none situation. Providing people with some elements of the service is better than providing no services. The best should not be made the enemy of the good. Services should be built up as resources which become available according to the level of need and the demand nor should integration result in dilution of available resources. Rather, it should result in more effective and optimum utilization of resources that are integrated.

Moreover, the integration between education and reproductive health care is two-directional. Education of girls is closely related to improvements in the health status of the family and the falling fertility rates. In turn, girls born into smaller families are more likely to be sent to school and to complete more years of schooling. Education of girls benefits the whole society. It has a more significant impact on poverty and development than the education of boys. It is also the most influencing factor in reducing maternal and infant mortality rates and improving the health and well being of generations.

Thus, there is a strongly felt need for public health community programmes to identify, prepare, integrate and implement maternal and child health care services that would help to promote health and healthy lifestyles of young women and their children and also to establish the mechanisms for delivery of population-based interventions along with their impact assessment. There is also a need to generate good quality and robust population data that can drive policies and programmes. Strategic investments in health, nutrition, education, empowerment and welfare of women are critical for healthy growth of young generation and these programmes need to be monitored and evaluated for their efficacy and effectiveness using public health approaches.

HOW THIS BOOK IS ORGANIZED

This book is organized into eight chapters. A brief description of each of its chapter follows:

Chapter 1 introduces the readers to the numerous implications for the health of women in the reproductive age group. It focuses on the specific health needs of women related to their sexual and reproductive functions.

This chapter gives an overview of global scenario as well as the regional status of women in reproductive age group so as to recognize the need for intervention strategies to promote healthy reproductive life of mothers and their offspring's. It also assesses the impact of reproductive health on the newborn which is immediate and can be dramatic. The magnitude of the burden of diseases, their impact and the glaring inequities are not enough to provide a rational basis for allocation of resources. The availability of cost-effective interventions has also to be considered.

Chapter 2 explains the anatomy, physiology and endocrinology of a normal pregnancy. The reproductive system, in function, dysfunction and disease, plays a crucial role in women's health. This is different from the case with men. A major burden of the disease in females is related to their reproductive system and their reproductive function and the way society treats or mistreats them because of their gender. Women, healthy women, need adequate health care in order to be able to carry their sexual/ reproductive functions and to carry them safely and successfully.

Chapter 3 focuses on the essentials of a normal healthy pregnancy so as to enable women to give birth to healthy children. This chapter provides information on lifestyle choices to maximize health throughout pregnancy and give the baby the best possible start in life. It includes guidelines on eating healthy, avoiding health hazards and dealing with disorders and illnesses. The problem of under-nutrition runs in generations and is dependent on multifarious factors which include proper infant and young child feeding practices, completion of immunization schedule, institutional delivery as far as possible, regular check-ups for early detection of childhood developmental delays and subsequent follow up, consumption pattern in families affecting the life of adults and elderly. Food fortification (salt iodization, enrichment of flours etc.), regular administration of deworming drugs, iron supplement to target the problem of iron deficiency anaemia and an access to safe drinking water and proper sanitation have overriding effects on the overall status on the nutritional attainment in commensurate with the ages and the physiological states such as pregnancy and lactation.

Chapter 4 deals with the identification of high risk pregnancies and the general risk factors contributing to these high risk pregnancies. Some women experience health problems or complications during pregnancy. These complications can adversely affect the mother's health, the fetus's health or of both of them. Even women, who were healthy before getting pregnant, can experience various complications. These complications may make the pregnancy a high-risk pregnancy. The risks of neglecting sexual and reproductive health of girls and women are great; a painful or damaging transition from adolescence to adulthood can result in a lifetime of ill effects. For girls, early pregnancy/ motherhood can be physically risky and can compromise their educational achievements and economic potential. Adolescent girls, in particular, face an increased risk of exposure to HIV/ AIDS and other Sexually Transmitted Infections (STIs), sexual coercion, sexual exploitation and violence. All of these have a huge impact on an individual's physical and mental health as well as long term implications for them, their offspring's, their families and their communities.

Chapter 5 explains the various concerns and complications of pregnancy. Complications of pregnancy are the health problems that are caused during pregnancy which make it a high risk pregnancy. Though most of the pregnancies go without any complication, still some women who are pregnant, experience complications that can involve their own health, their baby's health or both. Sometimes, diseases or conditions the mother had before she became pregnant can lead to complications during pregnancy. Some complications may also occur during the labour and delivery. Even with the complications of pregnancy, early detection and prenatal care can reduce any further risk to the mother and the baby.

Chapter 6 focuses on the obstetric labor complications of pregnancy. Complications that occur primarily during childbirth are termed obstetric labor complications. An obstetric labor complication is a difficulty or abnormality that arises during the process of labor or delivery. The second stage of labour may be delayed or lengthy due to poor or uncoordinated uterine action, an abnormal uterine position such as breech or shoulder dystocia and cephalo-pelvic disproportion (a small pelvis or large infant). Prolonged labour may result in maternal exhaustion, fetal distress and other complications, including obstetric fistula which may ultimately lead to maternal or neonatal mortality.

Chapter 7 highlights the problems and disorders that occur primarily after childbirth and are termed as puerperal disorders. A puerperal disorder or postpartum disorder is a disorder which presents primarily during the puerperium or postpartum period. World Health Organization (WHO) describes the postpartum period as the most critical and yet the most neglected phase in the lives of mothers and babies; most maternal and newborn deaths occur during the postpartum period. In addition to affecting the mother's health, it can interfere with her ability to connect with and care for her baby and may cause the baby to have problems with sleeping, eating and behavior as he or she grows.

Chapter 8 deals with the management of high risk pregnancies. Identifying high-risk pregnancies is an important step for the design of intervention programmes. For reproductive health services to be woman-friendly there is need to recognize and respond to the continuum of reproductive health care needs, they have to see the woman behind the mother, they have to see women as ends and not means and they have to tailor their services according to women's needs and perceptions. Maternal and Child Health, Adolescent Sexual and Reproductive Health, family planning and other reproductive health care services should be placed under one managerial responsibility so as to ensure that all reproductive health needs of women are adequately met, that all health needs receive a relatively adequate allocation of resources, that all health care services are adequately linked and coordinated and wherever and whenever appropriate, these are well integrated.

However, with regard to the service-related barriers, poor health care systems for the sexual health, family planning and maternal health are common, with unmarried adolescent girls ignored in some cases, married adolescent girls in others and an overall deficiency of youth-friendly services. Lack of integration of services is also there where such services that might address counseling and family planning fail to include HIV/STI care, etc. Services may also be hampered by corruption and lack/erratic availability of supplies and equipment. Moreover, economic and physical accessibility restrict the adolescent girl's access to these services wherever they do exist.

The challenge, however, is that all countries should strive to make accessible these health care services through their primary health-care system, reproductive health to all individuals of appropriate ages as soon as possible but not later than the year 2030, as enshrined in the Sustainable Development Goals (SDG's) of United Nations.

To achieve this, women friendly clinics need to be widely established throughout the country and should achieve a universal coverage. Screening of all women, especially pregnant women, on regular basis could be an effective tool to evaluate and manage the existing complications and to avoid the occurrence of high-risk pregnancies. Moreover, strategies should be made to empower and involve women in decision making process that affects them and facilitates them with every opportunity for developing into a healthy mother and give birth to healthy off-springs. Offering such opportunities to the pregnant women gives them a chance to build a safe, happy, healthy and productive nation in the future.

The present manuscript is an attempt to sensitize women in the reproductive age group, adolescent girls, prospective mothers and caregivers to understand the reproductive health needs of women in general and pregnant women in particular so as to enable them to give birth to healthy children who grow up as productive and contributing members of the society. This manuscript will help the planners and policy makers to strategize various maternal and child health programmes, adolescent reproductive and sexual health programmes and interventions and assess the impact of various health care approaches through the health status of mothers and the newborn.

Sapna Nanda
Panjab University, India

REFERENCES

Fathalla, M. F. (1994). From family planning to reproductive health. In L. A. Mazur (Ed.), *Beyond the numbers-A reader on population, consumption and the environment* (pp. 143–149). Island Press.

Morris, J. L., & Rushwan, H. (2015). Adolescent Sexual and Reproductive Health: The Global Challenges. *International Journal of Gynaecology and Obstetrics: the Official Organ of the International Federation of Gynaecology and Obstetrics, 131*, S40–S42. doi:10.1016/j.ijgo.2015.02.006 PMID:26433504

Murray, C. J. L., & Lopez, A. D. (1996). *The global burden of disease-Summary*. Harvard University Press.

Sedgh, G., Finer, L. B., Bankole, A., Eilers, M. A., & Singh, S. (2015). Adolescent Pregnancy, Birth and Abortion Rates across Countries: Levels and Recent Trends. *Journal of Adolescent Health, 56*, 223-230.

World Bank. (1993). *World Development Report- Investing in Health*. Oxford University Press.

World Health Organization. (1998). *Fifty-first World Health assembly, 11-16 May 1998: Resolutions and decisions, annexes*. World Health Organization.

Acknowledgment

It gives me immense pleasure in expressing my deep sense of gratitude to Almighty God for His blessings, direction and guidance to undertake this project. This arduous task could not have been accomplished without my utmost faith in His divine power.

I express my profound sense of reverence to my mentor Dr. (Mrs.) R. Puri, Professor Emeritus, Foods & Nutrition and Associate Dean (Retd.), College Development Council, Panjab University, Chandigarh for her scholarly inspiration, professional guidance and erudition throughout the course of this project. Working under her able guidance had been a rich and valuable learning and rewarding experience. Besides her professional support, her love, affection and blessings and constant motivation have shaped my personality.

I must acknowledge the contributions of all professionals, researchers and scholars who have been working extensively in the area of maternal and child health. Their emerging research findings have enriched my knowledge domain and made my project meaningful and relevant in the light of contemporary researches.

I shall be failing in my duty if I do not express my heartfelt gratitude to the team of IGI Global Publishing of United States of America for their faith in my abilities that has been a steering force for the initiation and completion of this project. I immensely appreciate the relentless and unconditional support of Ms. Jan Travers, Ms. Carlee Nilphai and Ms. Maria Rohde, my Development Editors for providing me the best technical assistance, motivation, immediate feedback and reinforcement from time to time and special gratitude to Ms. Lindsay Wertman for successful completion of this project.

Acknowledgment

I deeply acknowledge the contributions of my family and friends who have always been a source of constant inspiration and constructive suggestions that paved the way for improving the quality of this manuscript. I feel deeply indebted to my husband Shri Deepak Nanda and children, Arjun, Dimple and Swati for supporting me both academically, technically and emotionally with their utmost patience and boosting my morale for the timely completion of this assignment.

Last but not the least, I express my immense gratitude to each and everyone who has rendered an unconditional support for the final presentation of this manuscript.

Sapna Nanda

Chapter 1
Reproductive Health of Women

ABSTRACT

The tragedy of maternal mortality in the developing world is not just a health concern; it should be recognized as a human rights issue. The theme for World Health Day for 1998 was "Pregnancy is Special; let's make it safe." When this theme was adopted by the World Health Assembly, it set a principle in the health policy. Pregnancy is not a disease. Pregnancy is special. Pregnancy, a privilege for a woman, is the means for human species to survive and propagate. When women risk their lives and health in order to give birth to a new life, they have a right to safe motherhood. Pregnancy should, thus, not compete for resources with the disease conditions. It is for these reasons of disease burden, an impact that transcends national boundaries as well as a deep concern about social injustice and inequity along with the availability of cost-effective interventions, that a major investment in reproductive healthcare is justified.

KEY FACTS

- Many of today's 1·2 billion adolescents (i.e. people, aged 10 to 19 years) were born around the turn of the millennium, when world leaders first pledged to achieve the Millennium Development Goals (MDGs) (United Nations, 2011).
- Each year, an estimated 16 million women, aged 15 to 19 years give births (World Health Organization, 2013) and a further million become mothers before the age of 15 years (Neal et al, 2012).

DOI: 10.4018/978-1-7998-4357-3.ch001

- About 1 in 50 women dying in developing countries from complications of pregnancy and unsafe abortion, about 35 times more than their counterparts in the developed countries (World Bank, 1993).
- These young people have benefitted from improvements associated with the MDG's including a 47 percent drop in maternal mortality between the years 1990 and 2010 (World Health Organization, 2012).
- However, studies of maternal mortality tend to calculate single mortality figures for women and girls of all ages.

INTRODUCTION

Being a woman has multiple implications for her own health. Thus, the health-related needs of women can, thus, be broadly classified into four categories (Fathalla, 1997). Firstly, women have specific health needs related to the functions of sex and reproduction. Secondly, even before menarche after menopause, women have an elaborate reproductive system that is vulnerable to dysfunction or disease. Thirdly, women are subjected to the same diseases of other body systems that can affect men. Because of genetic constitution, hormonal environment or gender-evolved lifestyle behavior, their patterns of disease often differ from those of men. Diseases of other body systems or their treatments may interact with the conditions of the reproductive system or its functions. Fourthly, because women are women, they are subjected to social distress which has a devastating impact on their physical, mental or social health.

Concept of Health

In the Constitution of the World Health Organization (WHO), health is defined as a state of complete physical, mental and social well-being and not merely the absence of disease or infirmity (WHO, 1948). This is consistent with the bio-psycho-social model of health, which considers physiological, psychological and social factors in health and illness as well as the interactions between these factors. It differs from the traditional medical model, which defines health as the absence of illness or disease and stresses the role of clinical diagnosis and intervention. The WHO definition explicitly links health with wellbeing, and conceptualizes health as a human right that requires physical and social resources to attain and maintain it. 'Wellbeing' refers to a positive state as opposed to neutral, framing health as a positive aspiration. The Ottawa charter of 1986 this definition which describes health as 'a resource for everyday life, not the object of living'. From this perspective, health is a means to live well, which highlights the link between health and participation in society (Martino, 2017).

Concept of Reproductive Health

In the context of this positive definition, reproductive health is a condition in which the reproductive processes are accomplished in a state of complete physical, mental and social well-being and is not merely the absence of disease or disorders of the reproductive system and its functions. Reproductive health is, thus, a state of complete physical, mental and social well-being (not merely the absence of disease or infirmity) in all matters related to the reproductive system and its functions and processes. Reproductive health is, thus, not just a concern during a woman's so-called "reproductive years", customarily defined as the age between 15 to 45 years. Rather, the reproductive health is a lifetime concern from infancy to old age (Pillsbury et al, 2000). Women, thus, need reproductive health care appropriate to their situations during entire lifecycle.

In addition, the concept of reproductive health is not limited to mothers nor is it limited to women of childbearing age. It recognizes the adolescents ' special health needs related to their sexual and reproductive capacity acquisition before they complete their adult social preparation. It also recognizes mature women beyond the period of childbearing, who still have significant health needs related to their reproductive system which they still carry and the cessation of ovarian functions. This concept also recognizes that the adult woman's health builds on the individual's health during childhood and adolescence.

Reproductive health, thus, implies that people have the ability to reproduce, to regulate their fertility and to practice and enjoy sexual relationships, apart from the absence of disease or infirmity. Every individual has the right to make his / her own sexual and reproductive health decisions. It implies that people have a satisfying and safe sex life, the ability to reproduce and the freedom to decide whether, when and how often. They need to be well informed and empowered to guard themselves against sexually transmitted infections. When women decide to have children, they need an access to services that can help them undergo a safe pregnancy, secure delivery and a healthy baby.

It finally implies that reproduction is carried to a successful outcome through infant and child survival, growth and healthy development (UNFPA, 2016).

Reproductive health is, thus, an integrated package. Women cannot be healthy if they have one reproductive health element and miss another. In addition, the diverse elements of reproductive health are strongly interrelated. Improvements in one reproductive health element can lead to potential improvements in other elements. Likewise, lack of improvement in one component of reproductive health can inhibit progress in other components.

In many societies, discrimination against girls and women begins as early as in infancy and decides their entire life course. During early childhood and adolescence, concerns related to nutrition, education and appropriate health care often arise. These concerns continue during reproductive years also which include family planning, sexually transmitted diseases (STD's) and reproductive tract infections, inadequate nutrition and care during pregnancy as well as the social status of women. Certain common concerns of old age are chronic infections and increasing concern about cervical and breast cancer, thereby resulting in high incidence of morbidity and mortality among them (UNFPA, 2000).

Unfortunately, in many developing countries, where more than half a million women die each year from pregnancy-related causes, including unsafe abortion, maternal mortality remains all too common. This is equivalent to about 1 in 50 women who die from complications of pregnancy and unsafe abortion in developing countries, about 35 times that of their counterparts in developed countries (World Bank, 1993).

A mother's death has extremely serious consequences, particularly for an infant or a young child. In developing countries, if the mother dies, there is a high risk that her children under the age of 5 years will also die, a likelihood in some places is as high as 50 percent (World Bank, 1993).

Thus, the circumstances in which a child is born largely determine not only whether it survives but the whole course of its life. Women's reproductive choices significantly impact both their own and their children's life prospects. Consequently, mother's age, spacing of births and care during pregnancy and delivery are important determinants of infant survival and progress through childhood (UNFPA, 2000).

The reproductive health of pregnant women has an immediate and dramatic impact on the health of the newborn (World Health Organization, 1996). An estimated 7.6 million perinatal deaths (stillbirths and first-week deaths) occur each year in developing countries (World Health Organization, 1996). In general, children born to adolescent mothers are at a disadvantage, given the physical and emotional immaturity of the mother due to the fact that having a child usually puts an end to her schooling. The risks are particularly high for the child if the mother is a young adolescent (12 to16 years of age), unmarried, poor or unwanted. The burden of birth to an adolescent mother is highest under all these prevailing conditions (World Bank, 1993).

There are high risks of neglecting Adolescent Sexual and Reproductive Health (ASRH); a painful or harmful transition to adulthood that can lead to ill effects throughout life. Early pregnancy / motherhood can be physically risky for girls and can jeopardize her educational achievement and the economic potential. In particular, adolescent girls face increased risk of HIV exposure and sexually transmitted infections (STIs), sexual coercion, exploitation and violence. All of these have an enormous impact on the physical and mental health of an individual and have long-term implications for adolescent themselves, their families and their communities (Morris and Rushwan, 2015).

Infants of adolescent mothers are also at high risk due to the adverse socio-economic conditions, which are typically more severe when the mother is an adolescent. Adolescent mothers are generally less able to provide her premature or low birth-weight infant with the compensatory care. Other adults in poor families are also less likely to be available or able to provide the support needed for the mother and the newborn (World Bank, 1993).

Nearly half of all deaths among children under the age of five years occur in their first month of life. The risk of death of an infant during the first year in the developing countries is 30 percent higher if born to a young mother than to an adult woman (Alan Guttmacher Institute, 1998).

Infants born to adolescent mothers, even if they survive, are more likely to be premature and low birth-weight. In developing countries, such survival risks are far greater under the given the conditions of poverty, poor nutrition and poor availability of medical care. In addition, risky sexual behaviors and problems with reproductive health during adolescence can have long-lasting consequences for their adulthood and for the subsequent generations. An impaired foetal growth, for example, is more common in pregnancies occurring before the age of 18 years and low birth weight is an important risk factor for adult-onset of diabetes (Norris et al, 2012).

Overall, improvements in adolescent health have not kept pace with those observed in children over the past five decades. Though mortality among 1 to 4-year-old children has declined by more than 80 percent over the past five decades, the adolescent mortality rates have improved from 41 to 48 percent (Viner et al., 2011).

In the Dominican Republic, pregnancy has become the leading cause of death among girls, especially adolescent girls, aged 15 to 19 years. In this age group, nearly one in four girls is either pregnant or has already given birth. Using peer education and counseling, a project supported by UNFPA aims to reduce rates of adolescent pregnancy and infection with STD and AIDS by raising awareness among young people about the health risks of unprotected sex. Adolescents are encouraged to postpone their first sexual encounter or remain faithful to one partner (UNFPA, 2000).

Moreover, many young women resort to abortions. Usually, in most countries, abortion is not legal, except under certain circumstances, thus making it clandestine and unsafe. According to the Guttmacher Institute, abortion rates are similar in countries where abortion is legal and in countries where it is illegal. In parts of the world where abortion is illegal, botched abortions still cause 8 to 11 percent of all maternal deaths which constitutes approximately 30,000 annually (Khazan, 2018).

Even where abortion is legal, due to social stigma and inaccessibility of health care services, many young women resort to unsafe abortions. Though reliable data is scarce, an estimated 70,000 deaths each year result from the approximately 20 million unsafe abortions that occur annually. There are many of such deaths among adolescent girls and young women (Tsui et al, 1997).

In many countries largely in Asia, Southeastern Europe, the Middle East and some parts of Africa, girls suffer from deep-seated cultural preference for sons. Though the sex ratio was skewed in only six countries in 1995, it has spread to 21 countries today with a skewed sex ratio favoring boys. This growth of gender imbalance in only two decades indicates a widespread acceptance of modern technology predicting the sex of the foetus (Brink, 2015).

Young girls are often neglected in many poor communities and are denied an access to education and health care. Parents in every continent are keener to send their sons to school and make them stay longer as compared to their daughters. In some countries, strong preference for male child has led to sex-selective abortion of female foetuses, and even female infanticide. This particular form of gender-based discrimination has been made possible by increased availability of reproductive technology such as amniocentesis and ultrasound, thereby resulting in a higher-than-normal male-to-female sex ratio, as in China, the Republic of Korea and also in India. Sex-determination testing is now banned by the laws in India and China. Nevertheless, at least 60 million girls are going "missing" in Asia alone due to this phenomenon (UNFPA, 2000).

There is a strong and negative impact of mother's education on infant and child mortality. With each additional year of schooling of mother, there is a decrease in the probability of losing one under five-year-old child by 6 percent. Women with primary schooling have 5 percent lesser chance to experience the loss of a child as compared to an uneducated mother (Badji, 2016). On the contrary, women with more years of schooling have children who are much more likely to survive during infancy. Better-educated women are also more likely to have a better say in decision-making of issues related to their marriages and family planning. Education not only equips them with adequate knowledge that allows them to navigate their pregnancy but also has the potential to enable them to take control of their reproductive health and wellbeing (Sperling & Winthrop, 2015).

Unwanted pregnancy resulting in high levels of unsafe abortion is one major outcome of unmet need for family planning. Pregnancy and childbirth related complications are the leading cause of death among girls, aged 15 to 19 years in LMIC's where nearly all of the estimated 3 million unsafe abortions occur (Chandra-Mouli et al, 2014). Mostly as a result of unintended pregnancy, almost 4.5 million adolescent girls undergo an abortion every year worldwide, with around 40 percent abortions performed under unsafe conditions (Grimes et al, 2006).

Adolescent girls, who have ever had sex or are currently sexually active, are more likely than boys in the same categories to be or have been married (World Health Organization, 2007). Married adolescents usually don't want to be pregnant but have low rates of contraception. Indeed, the recent data revealed that current use of contraceptives among sexually active, married adolescents is often lower (Blanc et al, 2009). For example, in Bangladesh, the contraceptive use among women, aged 10 to 49 years, rose from 49 to 61 percent during the years 1996 to 2011 while for married adolescents, aged 15 to 19 years, it rose from 33 to 47 percent in the same time period (United Nations, 2013). Similarly, in Malawi, contraceptive use among married women, aged 15 to 49 years, increased from 13 to 46 percent during the years 1992 to 2010 whereas among married adolescents, aged 15 to19 years, it rose from 7 to 29 percent (United Nations, 2013). Unmet need for both married and unmarried adolescents is, therefore, still extremely high (Chandra-Mouli et al, 2014).

The unmarried adolescent girls on getting pregnant face three alternatives. She may marry her father; she will most likely drop out, if she is in school. The marriage and pregnancy may be unwanted and may soon lead to divorce or abandonment. A second and increasingly common alternative is that she can develop into a single mother, usually facing social disapproval and economic hardship. Thirdly, she could have an abortion, which is typically illegal and unsafe. However, if she undergoes pregnancy, there is a much greater risk of complications or dying during childbirth than if she had delayed childbirth until she was physically mature. Adolescent girls, aged 15 to 19 years, are five times more likely to die during pregnancy or childbirth as compared to older women, aged 20 to 24 years; the risk is even greater for younger girls. Various research studies in Chile, Mexico and the Caribbean reveal that adolescent mothers will have more children than those who begin childbearing later and will live more often and for longer periods with their parents or other family members. Fewer fathers of children will be heading the household or providing financial and other support (UNFPA, 2000).

Global Scenario of Reproductive Health

Maternal mortality is a significant global concern. Though a marked decrease in maternal mortality rate occurred in the United States during the mid-20th century, this progress was stalled during the late 20th century. In addition, rates of maternal mortality (MMR) have risen during the early 21st century. The maternal mortality rates began to rise around the year 2000 and have doubled since almost. Given that at least half of maternal deaths are preventable in the United States, the rise in maternal deaths in the United States is both historic and worrisome. The number of maternal deaths in United States has steadily increased to a high of 17.8 deaths per 1, 00,000 live births from the year 1987 to the year 2011. The reasons for the overall increase in maternal mortality rate are not clear (Neggers, 2016).

In most of the developing countries, more than half a million women die every year from pregnancy-related complications. There are four important reasons for maternal mortality and morbidity which include that births are either "too soon, too close, too many or too late". Maternal deaths are the tip of iceberg in these countries, signaling the daily tragedies of women's lives and reflecting how poverty in the world has been feminized. A woman dies every single minute. Every day approximately 1400 die and 0.6 million die in one year. Eighty percent die from pregnancy and childbirth complications and 99 percent of these deaths occur in Sub-Saharan Africa (SSA) and South Asia (WHO/ UNICEF / UNFPA, 2000). The United Nations estimated in 2003 that one in every 55 women in India face the risk of maternal mortality.

Maternal mortality is, thus, a very difficult medical, social, emotional and hence medico-legal situation, especially in third world countries.

The **Alma Ata** Declaration in 1978 stated that "The existing gross inequality in the health status of the people particularly between developed and developing countries as well as within countries is politically, socially and economically unacceptable and is, therefore, of common concern to all countries" (World Health Organization, 1978). Recently in the year 2018, 2000 delegates from more than 120 countries renewed the commitment with the Astana declaration for providing comprehensive primary health care for all. The new declaration on primary health care affirms that the "commitment to the fundamental right of every human being to the enjoyment of the highest attainable standard of health without distinction of any kind", and reaffirms its commitment to the core principles of Alma-Ata (WHO, 2019).

It has been recognized in the Astana Declaration that remaining healthy is challenging for many people, particularly the poor. It states that it is "unacceptable that inequity in health and disparities in health outcomes persist". Astana' is committed to prioritize disease prevention and health promotion as well as and aims at meeting the health needs of all people throughout life through its comprehensive preventive, promotional, curative, rehabilitative and palliative care services. The new Astana Declaration acknowledges the growing importance of non-communicable diseases, including mental health issues, injuries and climate change health impacts. In addition, Astana includes ' Universal Health Coverage,' which is at the heart of the Sustainable Development Goal (SDG) 3 (O'Connell, 2014). The SDG's (2015) succeeding the MDGs provides an impetus to the Alma Ata as well as Astana principles through other SDG's such as 'Equity' (SDG 10), 'Community Participation' (SDG 6) and 'Inter-sectoral Collaboration' (SDG 17). Evidence indicates that countries reorienting their health systems towards primary health care are better in a position to achieve almost all of the SDGs, including SDG 1 – 'To end poverty' (Pettigrew, 2015; Hone, 2018).

There is no health area in which inequity is as striking as it is in the reproductive health sector. Looking at the world's mortality differentials, it is found that while in the less developed regions, the crude death rate for the population is about ten percent higher than in the more developed regions, infant mortality rates are nearly six times higher, child mortality rates are seven times higher and maternal mortality rates are fifteen times higher. Mortality differentials in no area of public health are more marked than in maternal mortality (Fathalla, 1993).

The magnitude of the disease burden, its impact and glaring inequity are not sufficient to provide a rational basis for resource allocation. It also has to consider the availability of cost-effective interventions. While the total disability-adjusted lifeyears loss was almost the same for men and women in the 15 to 44-year-old age group, the percentage to be substantially controlled with cost-effective interventions was estimated at 43.9 per cent for women's diseases in comparison to 17.5 per cent for men's diseases (World Bank, 1993).

Moreover, in most societies, the psychological and social burden of infertility falls heavier on women. A social status of a woman is usually identified with her fertility and the failure to have children is viewed as a social disgrace or a reason for divorce. Thus, the sufferings of the infertile woman are very real. The female partner's infertility investigation is more elaborate and associated with more inconvenience and risk to her health. Also, the treatment burden mostly falls on the female partner. Even for male infertility, the promise of successful management is now shifting to the technologies of assisted conception, where the major burden is borne by female. The couple should, thus, commonly share the responsibility for infertility.

An analysis of data compiled in a large World Health Organization's multinational study on infertility also showed that a major factor in the female was diagnosed in only 12.8 percent of cases, with no demonstrable cause in the male. Whereas a major factor in the male was diagnosed in only 7.5 percent of cases, with no demonstrable cause in the female (World Health Organization, 1987). However, for biological and social reasons, the burden of infertility is unequally shared.

For a blend of biological and social reasons, women are, thus, more likely to be infected, are less likely to seek care, are more difficult to diagnose, are at higher risk of severe disease squealing, and are more likely to face social discrimination and consequences. Men control the most effective method available for protecting against STD's i.e. the condom. There is not yet a simple and effective method of protection which a woman can use without the need or necessity of the cooperation of her partner.

In the absence of a simple and effective method of protection, higher maternal mortality and morbidity rates of women are related to early childbearing (Blanc et al., 2013; Nove et al., 2014; Ganchimeg et al, 2014) and also to an increased risk of induced abortions, which are often illegal and unsafe (Shah & Åhman, 2012). Thus, the causes of maternal mortality and morbidity constitute the leading causes of death among adolescent females (WHO, 2011 a).

Complications resulting from pregnancy and childbirth are the leading cause of death globally for adolescent girls, aged 15 to 19 years. Worldwide, nearly 11 percent of all births happen to adolescent girls, aged 15 to 19 years and the vast majority of these births take place in low-and middle-income countries. Data analysis for the period 1985 to 2003 from 14 Latin American countries revealed that adolescent girls under the age of 16 years are four times more likely to die during pregnancy or childbirth than women between the ages of 20 and 24 years (Conde-Agudelo et al., 2005).

Adolescent pregnancy is, thus, associated independently with increased risks of low birth weight babies, premature delivery, severe neonatal conditions and early neonatal mortality due to an increased risk of premature birth (Ganchimeg et al, 2014). Of the estimated 22 million unsafe abortions occurring each year, 15 percent occur among young women, 15 to 19 years of age, and 26 percent occur among those, aged 20 to 24 years (WHO, 2011b).

A striking contrast between infant mortality rates for adolescent girls versus slightly older mothers was revealed through the data from Nigeria. For mothers who are under 20 years, infant mortality rate was 121 deaths per 1,000 live births in comparison to 79 deaths per 1,000 live births for the mothers, aged 20 to 29 years (World Bank, 1993).

Whatever the reasons for a baby being unwanted, it's likely that he or she will start life at a disadvantage. Abandonment is usual, a reason why street children in large cities from Manila to Rio de Janeiro are swelling in number. If the child is kept in the family, the mother may still not be prepared psychologically for child rearing responsibilities or resources of the family may not be adequate enough to meet the needs of the baby. The child is more likely to be abused (World Bank, 1993).

Regional Scenario of Reproductive Health

Sexual and reproductive health of adolescents is strongly associated with their particular social, cultural and economic environment. In addition to regional variation, experiences are diversified, among other features, by age, sex, marital status, schooling, residence, migration, sexual orientation and socio-economic status. An access to health care and educational, information and support sources also varies widely. Variations require pattern analysis at the country level but despite these variations, key issues, barriers and challenges as well as possible solutions need to be identified across the board (Morris and Rushwan, 2015).

Many adolescents become sexually active at an early age when they are unable to avoid unwanted pregnancies and infections that are sexually transmitted. Contextual or regional factors, such as pressure to conform to media stereotypes and their peers ' norms increase the chance of early and unprotected sexual activity (Nanda, 2019).

In September 2013, National Center for Health Statistics (NCHS) data from Centers for Disease Control and Prevention (CDC) confirmed a remarkable accomplishment; the United States adolescent birth rate decreased by 52 percent from its all-time high from 20 years ago (from 61.8 births in 1991 to 29.4 births in 2012 per 1,000 girls, aged 15 to 19 years) (Pearlman et al, 1990). In fact, the teen birth rates for all age groups and all racial/ethnic groups are now at historic lows since 1940's when National Center for Health Statistics (NCHS) started collecting data.

Despite this strikingly remarkable progress, United States still ranks the highest in adolescent births among higher-income countries, a burden aggravated further by persistent racial, economic and geographic disparities (Pearlman et al, 1990; Sammons, 1981).

Of note, more than 3,05,000 teens, aged 15 to 19 years, gave birth in the United States in the year 2012 (Pearlman et al, 1990). Furthermore, teen birthrates for Hispanics and non-Hispanic blacks are more than double that for non-Hispanic whites (Pearlman et al, 1990).

In most countries, these adolescent births are concentrated among poorer, less educated women and early motherhood further compounds the disadvantage by disrupting the school attendance and limiting their future livelihood opportunities. Context can vary considerably both between countries and within countries. In developing countries, most adolescent births are planned and occur within the context of marriage. These pregnancies are, therefore, driven by traditional practices and norms and promoted and sanctioned by families and the wider community (Nove et al, 2014).

In many African countries, pregnant adolescent girls are forced to leave the school and are also face moral persecution. For example, data from Rwanda reveal about 10 percent of pregnant school going adolescent girls being disowned by their families. This, in turn, can result in child abandonment ("baby dumping") and entry of the young mother into prostitution (World Bank, 1993).

Almost all community-based studies have suggested an increased risk of maternal mortality among adolescents in developing countries but estimates of the size of the increased risk vary greatly. In most developed countries, however, such as Latin America and the Caribbean and in some parts of

Sub-Saharan Africa (SSA), the majority of adolescent pregnancies occurs outside marriage and is often unplanned.

Studies from the developed countries are even less consistent: National estimates from the vital registration in the United States of America suggest that adolescents have a lower maternal mortality ratio than women older than 20 years (US Department of Health and Human Services, 2010). Statistics from the United Kingdom (Cantwell et al, 2011) and Canada (Health Canada, 2004), reveal that the maternal mortality ratio for women and girls younger than 20 years of age is slightly higher than for older women, aged 20 to 24 years but lower than those who older than 25 years.

On the other hand, Australian data suggest that the maternal mortality ratio for women under the age of 20 years is higher than that for all age groups other than women over the age of 40 years (Sullivan et al, 2008). Some evidence from both developing and developed countries also suggestive of the fact that younger adolescents are at higher risk, with girls aged 15 or younger, having higher mortality rates than their older counterparts (Conde-Agudelo et al, 2005).

Figures based on a United Nations report published more than 20 years ago (United Nations, 1991) indicate that adolescent girls, younger than 15 years of age, are five times and adolescent girls, between 15 to 19 years of age, are twice as likely to die from maternal causes as the older women. This report has only recently been challenged on the basis of a compilation of 13 datasets which suggests a reduced risk for the younger age group (Stover and Ross, 2009). An analysis of more recent data from 38 countries estimated that the risk of death per birth for adolescents, aged 15 to 19 years, is only 28 percent higher as compared to older women, aged 20 to 24 years (Blanc et al, 2013).

Thus, early-age first pregnancy is risky both for the mother's health as well as for the newborn. Although such births to adolescents account for 11 percent of all births worldwide, these account for 23 percent of the overall burden of DALY (in terms of disability-adjusted life years) diseases from pregnancy and childbirth among women of all ages (Patton et al, 2009).

The social consequences of pregnancy for adolescents include dropping out of school with subsequent lower educational achievement and reduced social opportunities, which include reduced earnings for life and violence, including suicide and homicide, in some settings (World Health Organization, 2012).

In low-and middle-income countries (LMIC's), pregnancy and childbirth related complications are the leading causes of death among women, aged 15 to 19 years. Adverse effects of childbearing on adolescents extend further to their infants ' health. In low-and middle-income countries (LMICs), stillbirths and deaths in the first week and first month of life are 50 percent higher among babies born to mothers younger than 20 years of age than those born to mothers, aged 20-29 years. The younger the mother, higher is the risk (Patton et al, 2009).

The potential health, social and economic disadvantages faced by adolescent mothers is widely recognized. Since the year 1990, their right to access to an adequate reproductive health care has been enshrined in a series of important international agreements and documents (UNICEF, 1990; United Nations, 1994; United Nations, 2011; United Nations, 2012). However, there is no accurate or comprehensive quantification of mortality risks to adolescent mothers. A commonly cited statistic indicate that adolescent girls younger than 15 years of age are several times at higher risk to die from maternal causes than women in their early 20's, (UNFPA, 2005) and those, aged 15 to 19 years, are also at an additional risk. (WHO, 2001; UN General Assembly, 2001).

The estimates of National Research Council and Institute of Medicine indicate 16 million births to mothers between the ages of 15 and 19 years, by 2008 worldwide. Around 95 per cent of these births take place in low- and middle-income (LMIC) countries (National Research Council and Medical Institute, 2005). Births to younger adolescents were relatively less common but one million births occur annually to girls, aged 12 to 15 years, according to recent estimates (Neal et al, 2012). While adolescent birth rates are declining, the absolute number of births has declined lesser due to an increase in adolescent population size (UNICEF, 2012).

The UN Population Division puts the global birth rate for adolescents at 44 births per 1000 adolescent girls in the year 2015. According to the Sustainable Development Goal (SDG) indicators, these age-wise variations in country rates range from 1 to over 200 births per 1000 adolescent girls. Those rates, however, indicate a marked decline from 1990. This decline is reflected in a similar decline in maternal mortality rates among adolescent girls, aged 15 to 19 years (United Nations, 1995).

Indian Scenario

In India, the fertility rate of adolescents contributing to the overall fertility rate by 17 percent and about 14 percent of births in women below 20 years of age are unplanned (Ministry of Health and Family Welfare, 2017). Early and unplanned risky adolescent pregnancies contribute to adverse pregnancy outcomes such as maternal mortality, babies with low birth weight, early neonatal deaths, eclampsia and congenital malformation (Ganchimeg, 2014).

Adolescents suffer from varied problems related to their sexual and reproductive health. As per National Family Health Survey (NFHS–3, 2005-06) data, 2.7 percent boys and 8 percent girls reported their sexual debut before age of 15 years and most of their sexual activity occurs in the context of marriage, thereby leading to an early pregnancy and its adverse effects. Although contraceptive awareness among adolescent girls between the ages of 15 and 19 years is 94 percent, only 23 percent of the married and 18 percent of the sexually active unmarried girls in this group used a contraceptive at least once (National Family Health Survey (NFHS-3), 2005–06).

All the findings of three NFHS surveys reveal nearly the same prevalence (59.1 percent, 59.8 percent and 58.2 percent) of pregnant and mothered adolescents. Over recent years, there is a steady rise in the percentage of first pregnancy among adolescents (11.7 percent, 12.4 percent and 14.4 percent) due to early marriage and low contraceptive use by pregnant adolescents (National Family Health Survey (NFHS-3), 2005–06).

However, exclusive data pertaining to the sexual and reproductive health issues of adolescent in Indian scenario is not available in comparison to other developing and developed countries. Nation and state-wise detailed investigations and reporting on adolescent's sexual and reproductive health issues is the need of the hour in order to create better awareness among the planners, policy makers as well as other stakeholders about the importance of strengthening adolescent sexual and reproductive health services under a single agency in order to meet their sexual and reproductive health needs.

Addressing current adolescent health issues can strengthen any nation not only today but tomorrow and further beyond. Because of the pressing emotional, social, health and financial consequences for both parents and their children, prevention of adolescent pregnancy, in particular, should rank as a major priority. The stakes are, no doubt, considerably high. Adolescent girls, who have babies are less likely to finish their high school or attend college; more likely to rely on public assistance; and more likely to live in poverty as adults as compared to those adolescents who delay childbearing.

In addition, children born to teens are more likely to have poorer long-term outcomes in terms of education, behavior and health as compared to children born to older parents (Hoffman, 2008). Overall, childbearing by teens costs billions of dollars to US taxpayers due to loss of tax revenue, higher payments for public assistance and higher spending on public health, foster care as well as criminal justice services (Hoffman, 2008; Hamilton et al., 2012).

In the year 2010, Teen Pregnancy Prevention (TPP) Program was launched by U.S. Department of Health and Human Services (HHS) with a central focus for the newly established Office of Adolescent Health (OAH). HHS Secretary Kathleen Sebelius called for implementing the best evidence-based initiatives in communities so as to maximize this new opportunity for teen pregnancy prevention, while also testing the new approaches (Koh, 2014).

Sexual and Reproductive Health Rights of Women

An access to comprehensive sexual and reproductive health and rights is a fundamental human right. The global status of the sexual and reproductive health and rights of women and girls, however, is worrying. Around 214 million women around the world want contraception, but lack access to it; more than 800 women die daily from causes of pregnancy and childbirth which are preventable; and same-sex relationships between consenting adults are still illegal in 76 countries worldwide (Global Fund for Women, 2020).

Globally, women and girls, especially those living in poverty, have either restricted or no access to information and services about their reproductive health and sexual rights. Discrimination, stigma, restrictive laws and policies, and entrenched traditions are some of the barriers to sexual and reproductive health and sexual rights. Despite the evidence that reproductive health and sexual rights have a transformative effect, not only on individual women, but on their families, communities and national economies, the progress remains slow. In order to drive equality with regard to the sexual and reproductive health and rights of all women, girls and trans-people must be fully and actively committed (Global Fund for Women, 2020).

Global Fund for Women believes that the ability of a woman to access comprehensive sexuality education, control her own body, and access the health services she needs, regardless of where she lives, her income level, or her ethnicity, is a basic fundamental right. In addition, all women, girls and LGBT people have the right to live without fear of violence or discrimination and should be able to make the best decisions for them about their sexuality and the sexual health (Global Fund for Women, 2020).

Sexual and Reproductive Health and Rights of LGBT

Lesbian, Gay, Bisexual and Transgender (LGBT) people across the globe continue to face endemic violence, legal discrimination and other violations of human rights because of their sexual orientation or gender identity. At least 76 countries around the globe (home to 44 per cent of the world's population) continue to criminalize same-sex relationships. Six countries (Mauritania, Sudan, Iran, Saudi Arabia, Yemen and Iraq) apply death penalty for same-sex relations, as do certain provinces in Nigeria and Somalia (Amnesty International, 2020).

Transgender Europeans also achieved significant triumphs over the recent years. Recently, Denmark became the first European country by allowing transgender people to obtain official documents reflecting their gender identity, without the need to be diagnosed with a mental disorder or undergo surgeries, thus resulting in an irreversible sterilization. More recently, Malta passed even more comprehensive law, thereby guaranteeing transgender and inter-sex human rights, recognizing that "gender identity is considered to be an inherent part of a person which may or may not need surgical or hormonal treatment or therapy" and that "sex characteristics of a person vary in nature and all persons must be empowered to make their decisions affecting their own bodily integrity and physical autonomy" (Amnesty International, 2020).

As we move from the International Day against Homophobia, Transphobia and Biphobia to mark pride across the United States, Amnesty International reaffirms the core conviction that all people, regardless of their sexual orientation or gender identity, should be able to exercise their full human rights in full solidarity with LGBT people whose fundamental rights are in jeopardy. The Supreme Court of India has taken proactive action, recognizing transgender people as a legal third gender and granting transgender Indians the status as an official minority, thus requiring protection against discrimination (Amnesty International, 2020).

CONCLUSION

For reproductive health care services to be woman-friendly, there is need to recognize and respond to the continuum of reproductive health care needs during entire life span, to see the woman behind the mother, to see women as ends and not as means as well as to tailor the reproductive health care services according to women's needs and perceptions.

REFERENCES

Alan Guttmacher Institute. (1998). *Into a new world: Young women's sexual and reproductive lives*. The Alan Guttmacher Institute.

Amnesty International. (2020). *The state of LGBT human rights Worldwide*. Retrieved from https://www.amnestyusa.org/the-state-of-lgbt-rights-worldwide/

Badji, S. (2016). *Mother's Education and Increased Child Survival in Madagascar: What Can We Say?* Academic Press.

Blanc, A. K., Winfrey, W., & Ross, J. (2013). New Findings for maternal mortality age patterns: Aggregated results for 38 countries. *PLoS One*, 8.

Brink, S. (2015). *Selecting Boys Over Girls Is Aa Trend In More and More Countries*. Retrieved from https://www.npr.org/sections/goatsandsoda/2015/08/26/434616512/selecting-boys-over-girls-is-a-trend-in-more-and-more-countries

Cantwell, R., Clutton-Brock, T., & Cooper, G. (2011). Saving mothers' lives: Reviewing maternal deaths to make motherhood safer: 2006–08. The eighth report on confidential enquiries into maternal deaths in the United Kingdom. *British Journal of Obstetrics and Gynaecology*, *118*(1), 1–203. PMID:21197681

Conde-Agudelo, A., Belizán, J. M., & Lammers, C. (2005). Maternal-perinatal morbidity and mortality associated with adolescent pregnancy in Latin America: Cross-sectional study. *American Journal of Obstetrics and Gynecology*, *192*(2), 342–349. doi:10.1016/j.ajog.2004.10.593 PMID:15695970

Crinson, I. (2007). *4a - Concepts of Health*. Wellbeing and Illness, and the Aetiology of Illness.

Diczfalusy, E., Griffin, P. D., & Khanna, J. (Eds.), *In: Research in Human Reproduction: Biennial Report (1986-1987)* (Vol. 341). World Health Organization.

Fathalla, M.F. (1988). *Research needs in human reproduction*. Academic Press.

Fathalla, M. F. (1993). The tragedy of maternal mortality in developing countries: A health problem or a human rights issue? *NU Nyttom U-landshalsovard*, *7*, 4–6.

Fathalla, M. F. (1996). Safe motherhood and child survival: The importance of family planning and the interdependence of services. In *Family Planning, Health and Family Well-being. Proceedings of the United Nations Expert Group Meeting on Family Planning, Health and Family Well-being, Bangalore, 26-30 October 1992*. United Nations, Department for Economic and Social Information and Policy Analysis-Population Division. New York. ST/ESA.R/131.

Fathalla, M. F. (1997). From obstetrics and gynecology to women's health-The road ahead. Parthenon publishing group.

Ganchimeg, T., Ota, E., Morisaki, N., Laopaiboon, M., Lumbiganon, P., Zhang, J., Yamdamsuren, B., Temmerman, M., Say, L., Tunçalp, Ö., Vogel, J. P., Souza, J. P., & Mori, R. (2014). Pregnancy and childbirth outcomes among adolescent mothers: A World Health Organization multi-country study. *British Journal of Obstetrics and Gynaecology*, *121*(1), 40–48. doi:10.1111/1471-0528.12630 PMID:24641534

Global Fund for Women. (2020). *Global Fund for Women Champions for Equality*. Retrieved from https://www.globalfundforwomen.org/sexual-reproductive-health-rights/

Hamilton, B. E., Martin, J. A., & Ventura, S. J. (2012). *Births: Preliminary data for 2011. National vital statistics report*. National Center for Health Statistics. Available at https://www.cdc.gov/nchs/data/nvsr/nvsr61/nvsr61_05.pdf

Health Canada. (2004). Special report on maternal mortality and severe morbidity in Canada—enhanced surveillance: the path to prevention. Ottawa: Minister of Public Works and Government Services, Canada.

Hoffman, S. D. (2008). Consequences of teen childbearing for mothers: Updated estimates of the consequences of teen childbearing for mothers. In Kids having kids: Economic costs and social consequences of teen pregnancy (2nd ed.). Washington, DC: Urban Institute Press.

Hone, T., Macinko, J., & Millett, C. (2018). Revisiting Alma-Ata: What is the role of primary health care in achieving the Sustainable Development Goals? *Lancet*, *392*(10156), 1461–1472. doi:10.1016/S0140-6736(18)31829-4 PMID:30343860

Khazan, O. (2018). *When Abortion Is Illegal, Women Rarely Die. But They Still Suffer*. Retrieved from https://www.theatlantic.com/health/archive/2018/10/how-many-women-die-illegal-abortions/572638/

Koh, H. (2014). The Teen Pregnancy Prevention program: An Evidence-Based Public Health Program Model. *The Journal of Adolescent Health, 54*(3), S1–S2. doi:10.1016/j.jadohealth.2013.12.031 PMID:24560068

Ministry of Health and Family Welfare. (2017). *Annual Report of Ministry of Health and Family Welfare 2014-15*. Government of India.

Morris, J. L., & Rushwan, H. (2015). Adolescent Sexual and Reproductive Health: The Global Challenges. *International Journal of Gynaecology and Obstetrics: the Official Organ of the International Federation of Gynaecology and Obstetrics, 131*, S40–S42. doi:10.1016/j.ijgo.2015.02.006 PMID:26433504

Murray, C. J. L., & Lopez, A. D. (1996). *The global burden of disease-Summary*. Harvard University Press.

Nanda, S. (2019). *Psycho-Socio-Physical Dimensions of Adolescent Health Management: Emerging Research and Opportunities*. IGI Global. doi:10.4018/978-1-5225-7384-5

National Family Health Survey (NFHS-3). (2005–06): India: Volume I. International Institute for Population Sciences (IIPS) and Macro International. (2007). Mumbai: IIPS. Available from: http://www.rchiips.org/nfhs/NFHS-3%20Data/VOL- 1/India_volume_I_corrected_17oct08.pdf

National Research Council. (2005). *Growing up global: The changing transitions to adulthood in developing countries*. The National Academies Press.

Neal, S., Matthews, Z., Frost, M., Fogstad, H., Camacho, A. V., & Laski, L. (2012). Childbearing in adolescents aged 12–15 years in developing countries: A neglected issue. New estimates from demographic and household surveys in 42 countries. *Acta Obstetricia et Gynecologica Scandinavica, 91*(9), 1114–1118. doi:10.1111/j.1600-0412.2012.01467.x PMID:22620274

Neggers, Y. H. (2016). Trends in Maternal Mortality in United States. *Reproductive Toxiology, 64*(9), 72–76. doi:10.1016/j.reprotox.2016.04.001 PMID:27063184

Norris, S. A., Osmond, C., Gigante, D., Kuzawa, C. W., Ramakrishnan, L., Lee, N. R., Ramirez-Zea, M., Richter, L. M., Stein, A. D., Tandon, N., & Fall, C. H. D. (2012). Size at birth, weight gain in infancy and childhood, and adult diabetes risk in five low- or middle-income country birth cohorts. *Diabetes Care*, *35*(1), 72–79. doi:10.2337/dc11-0456 PMID:22100968

Nove, A., Matthews, Z., Neal, S., & Camacho, A. V. (2014). Maternal mortality in adolescents compared with women of other ages: Evidence from 144 countries. *The Lancet. Global Health*, *2*(3), e155–e164. doi:10.1016/S2214-109X(13)70179-7 PMID:25102848

O'Connell, T., Rasanathan, K. & Chopra, M. (2014).What does universal health coverage mean? *Lancet*, *383*, 277-9. doi:8 doi:10.1016/S0140-6736(13)60955-1

Patton, G. C., Coffey, C., Sawyer, S. M., Viner, R. M., Haller, D. M., Bose, K., Vos, T., Ferguson, J., & Mathers, C. D. (2009). Global patterns of mortality in young People: A systematic analysis of population data. *Lancet*, *374*(9693), 881–892. doi:10.1016/S0140-6736(09)60741-8 PMID:19748397

Pearlman, M. D., Tintinalli, J. E., & Lorenz, R. P. (1990). Blunt trauma during pregnancy. *The New England Journal of Medicine*, *323*(23), 1609–1613. doi:10.1056/NEJM199012063232307 PMID:2233950

Pettigrew, L. M., De Maeseneer, J., Anderson, M. I., Essuman, A., Kidd, M. R., & Haines, A. (2015). Primary health care and the Sustainable Development Goals. *Lancet*, *386*(10009), 2119–2121. doi:10.1016/S0140-6736(15)00949-6 PMID:26638948

Pillsbury, B. L. K., Maynard-Tucker, G., & Nguyen, F. (2000). *Women's Empowerment and Reproductive Health: Links throughout the Life Cycle*. Academic Press.

Sammons, M.N. (1981). Battered and pregnant. *The American Journal of Maternal/ Child Nursing, 6*, 246-50.

Shah, I. H., & Åhman, E. (2012). Unsafe abortion differentials in 2008 by age and developing country region: High burden among young women. *Reproductive Health Matters*, *20*(39), 169–173. doi:10.1016/S0968-8080(12)39598-0 PMID:22789095

Sperling, G. B., & Winthrop, R. (2015). *What works in girls' education: Evidence for the world's best investment*. Brookings Institution Press.

Stover, J., & Ross, J. (2009). How increased contraceptive use has reduced maternal mortality. *Maternal and Child Health Journal, 14*(5), 687–695. doi:10.100710995-009-0505-y PMID:19644742

Sullivan, E., Hall, B., & King, J. (2008). *Maternal deaths in Australia 2003–2005*. Australian Institute of Health and Welfare.

Tsui, A. O., Wasserheit, J. N., & Haaga, J. g. (1997). *Reproductive Health in Developing Countries: Expanding Dimensions, Building Solutions*. National Academic Press.

UNFPA. (2000). *Women Empowerment and Reproductive Health: Links throughout the Life Cycle*. United Nations Population Fund.

UNFPA. (2005). *State of world population 2005: the promise of equality*. United Nations Population Fund.

UNFPA. (2016). *Sexual and Reproductive Health*. Retrieved from https://www.unfpa.org/sexual-reproductive-health

UNICEF. (1990). The United Nations Convention on the Rights of the Child. UNICEF.

United Nations. (1991). The world's women, 1970–1990: Trends and statistics. New York: UN.

United Nations. (1994). *UN Population Information Network*. Report of the International Conference on Population and Development, Cairo, Egypt.

United Nations. (1995). *Population and development: Programme of action adopted at the International Conference on Population and Development*. Dept. for Economic and Social Information and Policy Analysis.

United Nations. (2011). The Millennium Development Goals report 2011. New York: UN.

United Nations. (2011). UN Department of Economic and Social Affairs. In World population prospects: the 2010 revision. New York: UN.

United Nations. (2012). UN Economic and Social Council. In *Commission on Population and Development: report on the forty-fifth session*. New York: UN.

United Nations General Assembly. (2001). *We the children: end-decade review of the follow-up to the World Summit for Children. Report of the Secretary-General. United Nations*. United Nations Population Fund.

US Department of Health and Human Services. (2010). *Women's health USA: Maternal mortality*. https://mchb.hrsa.gov/whusa10/hstat/mh/pages/237mm.html

Viner, R.M., Coffey, C., & Mathers, C. (2011). 50-Year mortality trends in children and young people: A study of 50 low-income, middle-income, and high-income countries. *Lancet, 377*, 1162-74.

WHO/UNICEF/UNFPA. (2000). *Estimates: Maternal Mortality in 2000.* Author.

World Bank. (1993). *World Development Report- Investing in Health.* Oxford University Press.

World Health Organization, Division of Reproductive Health. (1998). World Health Day 1998: Safe Motherhood: Information Kit. World Health Organization.

World Health Organization. (2001). *The second decade: Improving adolescent health and development.* World Health Organization.

World Health Organization. (2011a). *Preventing early pregnancy and poor reproductive outcomes among adolescents in developing countries.* World Health Organization.

World Health Organization. (2011b). *Mortality estimates by cause, age and sex for the year 2008.* World Health Organization.

World Health Organization. (2012). *WHO, UNICEF, UNFPA, World Bank. Trends in maternal mortality: 1990 to 2010.* World Health Organization.

World Health Organization. (2013). *Adolescent pregnancy.* https://www.who.int/maternal_child_adolescent/topics/maternal/adolescent_pregnancy/en/

World Health Organization. (2018). *Declaration of Astana.* Geneva: World Health Organization. Available: https://www.who.int/ primary-health/conference-phc/declaration

Chapter 2
Physiology of Pregnancy

ABSTRACT

Pregnancy is associated with profound anatomical, physiological, biochemical, and endocrine changes that affect multiple organs and systems. One fertilized egg cell implanted in the lining of uterus initiates countless bodily changes. Secretion of ovarian hormones increases greatly. The bone marrow produces more RBCs and blood volume increases. The heart enlarges slightly to handle an extra supply of blood and shifts its position as uterus enlarges with the growing fetus. Such changes are necessary to help women adapt to the pregnant state and to support the growth and survival of the fetus. Such anatomical and physiological changes can also create confusion during a pregnant woman's clinical review. Likewise, changes in the biochemistry of blood during pregnancy may cause difficulties in interpreting tests. Hence, there is need to understand the deviation from normal anatomical, physiological, biochemical, and endocrine changes occurring during pregnancy so as to plan appropriate strategies for better maternal and fetal health.

KEY FACTS

- The anatomical, physiological and biochemical adaptations that occur during pregnancy are profound and revert to the non-pregnant state after the child birth and lactation.
- Maternal adjustments are attributed to pregnancy hormones and the mechanical pressures exerted by the enlarged uterus and other tissues.

DOI: 10.4018/978-1-7998-4357-3.ch002

- Adaptations to pregnancy protect the normal physiological functioning of women, meet the metabolic requirements imposed by pregnancy and provide for the development and growth needs of fetuses.
- Some adaptations to pregnancy result in discomforts like nausea, fatigue, urinary frequency and breast sensitivity.
- Within a period of 280 days of pregnancy, the body of mother is almost totally transformed as it accommodates itself to the creation of a new life. Another transformation process begins as the body of the mother returns to its well-functioning non-pregnant state.

INTRODUCTION

The reproductive system plays a central role in the overall health status of females in function, dysfunction and disease. This is different from the men's case though. A major burden of the disease in females is related to their reproductive system and reproductive function and how they are treated or mistreated by society due to their differential gender.

While more men die as a result of what one might call their "vices," women often suffer as a result of their nature-assigned physiological role in procreation and species survival, and related tasks. In a study reported by the World Bank on health investment, gender differential was shown in the ranking of the five main causes of the disease burden among young adults, aged 15 to 44 in the developing nations (World Bank, 1993).

Women, especially healthy women, need health care in order to be able to carry out their sexual/ reproductive functions safely and successfully. There has been a vast expansion of health technologies and health care services in the second half of this century to provide women with certain elements of reproductive health care.

However, those services were not without deficiencies. Besides inadequate resource allocation, the major shortcoming was in the philosophy with which these services were planned and provided. Women were seen as means in the reproductive process and as targets in the fertility control process. These services were not being provided as ends in themselves to women. Though the services benefited women, they were used as means and not as target beneficiaries.

The Biology of Pregnancy

Pregnancy is a unique state in both the mother's and the developing embryo's lifecycle. The resulting embryo, called the zygote, begins to divide and subdivide after egg and sperm unite within the oviduct. The embryo implants itself in the lining of the mother's uterus on the fifth or sixth day after fertilization. At this point, the placenta begins to form the specialized cells within the embryo. This organ connects the developing fetus to the mother and allows nutrients, gases, and waste to be exchanged. While there is no mixture of maternal and fetal blood in the placenta, the maternal blood vessels that underlie this organ are more dilated than normal to provide adequate oxygen and nutrients required to the growing foetus. The umbilical cord attaches the developing foetus to the placenta. During delivery, first the baby is delivered through the birth canal followed by the placenta (Government of Western Australia, Department of Health, 2019).

Oogenesis and spermatogenesis are two forms of reproductive divisions which are involved in human sexual reproduction. Reproductive division, also known as gametogenesis, occurs through meiosis in the germ cells in gonads. It's engaged in gametes production. The germ cell Diploid produces haploid gametes. There are two distinct groups of gametes: male gametes and female gametes. Male gametes are called sperm and eggs are known as female gametes. To form the diploid zygote, one sperm is combined with an egg, which undergoes division and differentiation to form a new organism. The key difference between spermatogenesis and oogenesis is that spermatogenesis is the process of sperm development from male germ cells and spermatogonia in males while oogenesis is the formation of eggs in females from female germ cells, oogonia (Panawala, 2017).

Oogenesis

Generation of female gametes, ova in the ovary from oogonia, is called oogenesis. The primary oocyte is the diploid cell, divided by meiosis, which forms a single ovum. Two polar bodies are formed, one at each of the two stages of meiosis. From puberty to menopause, oogensis occurs once a month. Oogenic germ cells, called oogonia, are stem cells, which are self-regenerating and differentiating into ova. During embryonic development, approximately 7 million germ cells are formed during the second to seventh months of the embryo through the division of thousands of oogonia. The primary oocytes are formed by mitosis from oogonia. During the embryonic phase, primary oocytes are processed until the diplotene stage of the initial meiotic division. The division of cells will be arrested, as it is before puberty. For around 50 years, certain primary oocytes have been arresting their cell division. Many of the primary oocytes are killed during lifetime and only about 400 primary oocytes eventually become gametes after puberty. Puberty begins the arrested division of cells, separating secondary oocyte from the primary oocyte. Here, the primary oocyte produces one secondary oocyte and one polar body by unequal division of the cells. The secondary oocyte contains the entire cytoplasm and the polar body nucleus is destroyed. During ovulation, secondary oocyte is released from the ovary (Panawala, 2017).

Spermatogenesis

The generation of male gametes, sperm, is called spermatogenesis which is produced from spermatogonia in the testis. The diploid cells form the spermatogonium. This can be located in the tiny testis tubules, which is the main reproductive organ of males. The spermatogonium is responsible for the four, haploid spermatozoa development. Cell division occurs by meiosis. Spermatogenesis begins with puberty in the males. Literally, for the rest of the males ' life, millions of sperms are produced per day. Spermatogonia are the spermatogenic germ cells. Spermatogonia is a stem cell that can regenerate itself. These differentiate into intermediate spermatogonium, which is dedicated to spermatozoa differentiation. Form B spermatogonia induces mitosis of the intermediate spermatogonium, which then undergoes mitosis, forming primary spermatocytes. Primary spermatozoa then undergoes meiosis 1, which produces two secondary spermatozoa. The resulting haploid cells are called spermatids which are still bound via cytoplasmic bridges to the boundary of the testis lumen. Spermatides are round, unflagellated cells which, during spermiogenesis, mature and differentiate into sperm. Human sperm production takes about 70 days to complete. Testis produces 100 million sperms a day in humans (Panawala, 2017).

Fertilization

Fertilization is the process through which gametes (an egg and sperm) fuse into a zygote form. The eggs and sperm each have a set of chromosomes. To ensure that the offspring has only one complete set of chromosomes, one sperm only needs to be fused with one egg. Fertilization is a process of cell-cell recognition that takes place between two distinct cells: a small asymmetric and mobile sperm cell, and a large, non-motile egg. The fertilization phases can be divided into four processes: 1) sperm preparation, 2) sperm-egg recognition and binding, 3) sperm-egg fusion, and 4) sperm and egg pronuclei fusion and zygote activation (Molnar and Gair, 2019).

As the cilia push the sperm towards the egg, the Fallopian tube pushes the egg toward the uterus. Progesterone and estrogen influence this process by increasing cilia counts and how quickly they move (Jones & Lopez, 2006). The egg and surrounding cells produce a chemical that attracts sperm (JOnes & Lopez, 2006; Moore et al, 2016). Sperm may be attracted to the temperature at the ovarian-end of the fallopian tube, which tends to be warmer (JOnes & Lopez, 2006; Suarez & Pacey,2006). As they travel through the fallopian tubes, sperms gain the ability to fertilize an egg (JOnes & Lopez, 2006). They undergo two processes: *capacitation*, where its outer layer is changed, and *hyperactivation*, which changes the way the sperm's tail moves (JOnes & Lopez, 2006; Suarez & Pacey,2006). Although it has come so far and has already changed, the sperm still has work to do: specifically, breaking through the barriers around the egg (Boutot, 2019).

Cleavage

The multi-cellular organism development begins with a single-celled zygote, which undergoes rapid cell division to form the blastula. The rapid, multiple cell division rounds are called cleavage. The embryo is named a blastula after the cleavage has produced over 100 cells. The blastula is usually a spherical layer of cells (the blastoderm) surrounding a cavity (the blastocoel) filled with fluid or yolk. At this stage, a structure called the blastocyst is formed which is characterized by an inner cell mass which is distinct from the surrounding blastula. The cells divide during cleavage without increasing the mass; that is, one large single-celled zygote divides into several smaller cells. Each cell within the blastula is called a blastomere (Molnar and Gair, 2019).

In the next stage of development, blastula forms the blastocyst. Here the blastula cells are arranged in two layers: the inner cell mass and an outer layer, called the trophoblast. Also known as the embryoblast, is the inner cell mass and that mass of cells will continue to form the embryo. At this stage of development, the inner cell mass consists of embryonic stem cells which differentiate the organism into the different cell types that it needs.

The trophoblast will aid the placenta and nourish the embryo (Molnar and Gair, 2019).

Implantation

The term "implantation" is used to describe the process of attachment and invasion by the blastocyst (conceptus) of the uterus endometrium. In humans, the process initiates at the end of first week, with most successful human pregnancies, the concept implants 8 to 10 days after ovulation but with later implantation, early pregnancy loss increases. The implantation process continues through the second week of development (Hill, 2020). The fertilized egg must attach to the uterus to become a viable pregnancy.

Placenta

The placenta is a temporary organ that begins to form shortly after implantation from the trophoblast layer of the cells. The placenta continues to develop and grow to satisfy the growing foetus ' needs. A fully developed placenta consists of a large mass of blood vessels, both from the mother and the foetus. The maternal and foetal vessels are close but separated by small spaces. This allows the blood of the mother and the foetus to exchange substances through their capillary walls without actually mixing the blood.

Through the umbilical cord, the foetus is connected to the placenta, a tube which contains two arteries and a vein. Blood from the foetus passes through the umbilical arteries into the placenta, exchange of gases and other substances takes place with the mother's blood and travels back to the foetus through the umbilical vein.

Development of the Foetus

this period is divided into three specified periods of three months each, making it nine months of pregnancy.

The First Trimester (0-3 Months)

The foetus is nearly 3.5 inches long by the end of the first trimester. The vital organs and the limbs are fully formed but not developed enough. During the first 12 weeks, the foetus is most vulnerable. All major organs and body systems are forming over this period of time and can be damaged, if the foetus is exposed to drugs, German measles, radiation, tobacco and chemical and toxic substances. Even though by the end of 12 weeks, the organs and body systems are fully formed, the foetus can't survive independently. The amniotic sac contains about 3.5 ounces of amniotic fluid and there is plenty of room for the foetus to move about, although the mother doesn't feel the movement.

By the end of first trimester, the foetus is about 3.5 inches long. The vital organs and the limbs are fully formed but not sufficiently developed. The foetus is most vulnerable during the first 12 weeks. During this period of time, all of the major organs and body systems are forming and can be damaged if the foetus is exposed to drugs, German measles, radiation, tobacco, and chemical and toxic substances. Even though the organs and body systems are fully formed by the end of 12 weeks, the foetus cannot survive independently. The amniotic sac contains about 3.5 ounces of amniotic fluid and the foetus has plenty of room to move about, although the movement is not felt by the mother. The heart begins to beat, facial features are fully formed and sex organs fully developed to identify foetus sex. The foetus swallows the amniotic fluid, its body uses most of it and it produces drops of sterile urine. The amniotic fluid in the amniotic sac is constantly refreshed. Since the foetus does not breathe independently, it does not suffocate. It gets the oxygen through the umbilical cord from the mother's bloodstream (Stanford children's health, 2020).

The Second Trimester (4-6 Months)

By the end of second trimester, the foetus is about 14 inches long and weighs about little less than one kilogram. The trunk and legs of the foetus lengthen and the head no longer looks too large for the rest of the body. At the beginning of second trimester, the mother begins to feel the movements of foetus. At the tip of fingers and toes, ridges develop, giving the foetus the unique identity of finger prints. Eyelashes and eyebrows appear though the eyes remain closed till the end of this trimester. The foetus now swallows a pint of amniotic fluid every day and returns it by urination to the amniotic sac. Every hour, the amniotic fluid is recycled when one-third of it is absorbed into the bloodstream of the mother and replaced by fresh fluid secreted from the amniotic sac.

The Third Trimester (7-9 Months)

Foetus is gaining weight during the last trimester and is growing in size. As it gets big, as it gets cramped for space, it can no longer move freely like before.

Now the mother feels its kicks instead of the foetus ' movements. During this trimester, the foetus store protein to build up their muscles, calcium for their bones, iron for their red blood cells and fat for insulation against changes in post-birth temperature.

By the end of seventh month in this trimester, the brain of the foetus matures to be able to cope up with the bodily functions of breathing and swallowing. If born at this stage, it has 90 percent chances of survival.

By the end of eight months, the foetus looks quite like what it looks at birth. Although the lungs are not fully functional, the foetus has 95 percent chances of survival if born at this stage. It is during the last trimester that the foetus opens its eyes; the sense organs undergo maximum development during this stage. Hairs grow on the head and the nails of fingers and toes also grow.

In general, the foetus turns his head down in the womb during the ninth month. It descends about two inches about two weeks before birth, settling in the pelvic bones of the mother. This is called lightening, enlargement or head fixing. As a result, the mother feels lighter as the foetus pressure pushing on her diaphragm and lungs are decreased so that she can breathe easier. In the ninth month, mild contractions of the womb muscles can be felt as the womb changes the foetus into the head-down position or the womb prepares its muscles for delivery. Sometimes however, the babies are born with feet first.

Anatomical and Physiological Adaptations in Mother

Pregnant women undergo profound anatomical and physiological changes so they can cope with their pregnancies ' increased physical and metabolic demands. The cardiovascular, respiratory, hematological, renal, gastrointestinal and endocrine systems all undergo significant physiological alterations and adaptations needed to enable the foetus to develop and allow the mother and fetus to survive the childbirth demands. Clinicians need to recognize pathological deviations in these normal anatomical and physiological changes during pregnancy to institute appropriate action to improve maternal and fetal outcome (Yanamandra and Chandraharan, 2012).

Such anatomical and physiological alterations / adaptations can cause difficulties in interpreting the signs, symptoms and biochemical investigations, making a pregnant woman's clinical assessment inevitably confusing but challenging. Understanding these changes is important for every practitioner, as pathological deviations from normal physiological changes may not be clear-cut until an adverse result has been achieved. Only a sound knowledge of the physiological and anatomical changes can safely optimize the care of an obstetric parturient for a better maternal and fetal outcome (KienTan and LoyTan, 2013).

Anatomy of Reproductive System

The pregnant mother undergoes significant anatomical and physiological changes during pregnancy in order to support and accommodate the developing foetus. After conception these changes start and affect every organ system in the body. For most women with an uncomplicated pregnancy, these changes resolve with limited residual effects after birth. It is important to understand the normal anatomical structure of reproductive system of women so as to understand the changes occurring during pregnancy as this will help to differentiate from adaptations that are not normal.

The Ovaries

The ovaries are paired, oval organs attached by the mesovarium (a fold of peritoneum, continuous with the outer surface of the ovaries) to the posterior surface of the broad uterus ligament. Neurovascular structures enter via the mesovarium into the ovary hilum. The main functions of the ovaries are to produce oocytes (female gametes) in preparation for fertilization and in response to pituitary gonadotrophins (LH and FSH), to produce the sex steroid hormones oestrogen and progesterone.

Each ovary measures about 35 mm in length, 25 mm in width and 18 mm in thickness. It is almond shaped and pearly grey with slightly corrugated surface. The ovary is attached by a thin mesentery, the mesovarium, to the back of the broad ligament. The ovary is laterally related to the fossa beneath the bifurcation of the common iliac artery and the ureter. Medially, it's close to the fimbria of the Fallopian tube, which stretches about ovulation over it. It is fixed by the ovarian ligament to the uterus cornu. The infundibulo-pelvic ligament is the outer order of the wide ligament and contains the ovarian vessels, nerves, and lymphatics. The ovary has 3 components. Simple cuboidal epithelium, known as germinal epithelium, forms the surface layer of the ovary. The cortex (outer part) of the ovary consists largely of a connective tissue, stroma which supports thousands of follicles. Each primordial follicle contains an oocyte which is surrounded by a single layer of follicular cells. The inner part, medulla, is composed of supporting stroma and contains a rich neurovascular network which enters the hilum of ovary from the mesovarium (Thompson, 2019).

The Fallopian Tubes

The fallopian tube measures 10 cm or more in length and approximately 4 mm in diameter which diminishes near the cornu of the uterus. Each fallopian tube is attached to the uterine cornu and its lumen is continuous with the cavity of the uterus. The fallopian tube is divided anatomically into four parts. The innermost part of the tube, **the interstitial portion**, traverses the myometrium to open into the endometrial cavity, is the narrowest portion and about 18 mm in length. There are no longitudinal muscle fibres but circular fibres are well developed. **The isthmus**, 35 mm long and with a lumen of 2 mm diameter and relatively straight, is the next and innermost part of the tube and represents about one-third of the total length. Its muscle wall contains both longitudinal and circular fibres. **The ampulla** is the lateral, widest and the longest part measuring 60-75 mm in length and comprises nearly two-third of the tube. **The fimbriated extremity or infundibulum** is where the abdominal ostium opens into the peritoneal cavity. The fimbriae are motile and show considerable range of movement and action. One fimbria, the ovarian fimbria, is larger and longer than the others and is attached to the ovary.

The Uterus

The uterus is approximately 9 cm long, 6.5 cm wide and 3.5 cm thick and is pyriform in shape. Anatomically and physiologically, it is divided into the body and the cervix. The fundus of the uterus lies above the insertion of the fallopian tubes and its cavity communicates with the opening of the fallopian tubes. The wall of the uterus has three layers, the peritoneal covering called perimetrium, the muscle layer or myometrium and the mucous membrane or endometrium.

The Cervix

The cervix is the lower portion of the uterus, a reproductive tract organ for females. It connects the vagina to the uterus ‘ main body, and acts as a gateway between them. The cervix is anatomically and histologically distinct from the uterus and thus it has a separate anatomical structure. Two regions comprise the cervix; the ectocervix and the endocervical canal. The ectocervix is the portion of the cervix that vaginally projects into it. It is lined with stratified, non-keratinized squamous epithelium. The outer os, the opening in the ectocervix, marks the transition from the ectocervix to the endocervical canal. The more proximally is the endocervical canal (or endocervix) and 'inner' part of the cervix. A mucus-secreting simple columnar epithelium lines it. The endocervical canal ends and the uterine cavity begins at a narrowing, that is called the internal os.

The two main functions of the cervix are to facilitate the passage of sperm into the uterine cavity achieved by dilating the external and internal os and maintaining the upper female reproductive tract's sterility. The cervix, along with all other structures superior to it, is sterile. By preventing bacterial invasion, this protects the uterine cavity and the upper genital tract ultimately. Frequent endometrial shedding, thick cervical mucus and a narrow outer os helps in maintaining this environment (Thompson, 2019).

Figure 1. Anatomical structure of a nulliparous uterus (Adapted from "Holland and Brew's Manual of Obstetrics", 16 Edn, 1998)

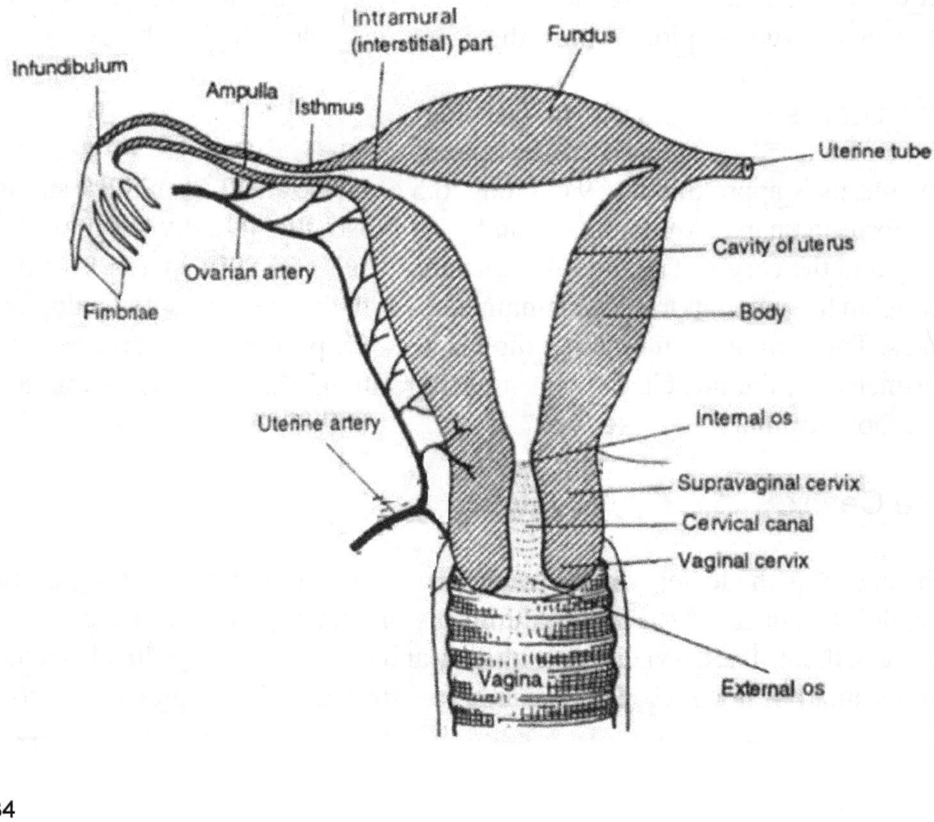

The Vagina

The vagina is a reproductive tract organ for females. The vagina is a muscle tube which distensible and extends to the cervix from the outer vaginal orifice to the postero-superior. The vagina is attached to the cervix at a higher level posteriorly and this makes the posterior vaginal wall longer than the anterior. The posterior vaginal wall is 11.5 cm long and the anterior wall is 9 cm long. The transverse folds on the vaginal wall allow the vagina to stretch and dilate during coitus and parturition. The anterior vaginal wall has three sulci; the submeatal sulcus, immediately above the meatus; the transverse vaginal sulcus, corresponding to the junction of urethera and bladder and the bladder sulcus, corresponding to the junction of bladder and anterior vaginal wall (Thompson, 2019).

The Vulva

The Vulva is bounded anteriorly by pubis, laterally by labia majora and posteriorly by the perineum. The labia majora consists of folds of skin which enclose a variable amount of fat and are best developed in the child bearing period of life. The labia majora are covered with squamous epithelium and contain sebaceous glands, sweat glands and hair follicles. The glands secrete a lubricating mucous during coitus. On the inner side of the labia majora lie the labia minora, the thin folds of skin which enclose veins and the elastic tissue but do not contain any sebaceous glands and hair follicles. The labia majora are erectile during sexual activity. Anteriorly, they enclose the clitoris and posteriorly join to form the fourchette, a thin fold of skin which is often torn during parturition.

Parturition means childbirth. Childbirth is the culmination of pregnancy, during which a baby grows inside a woman's uterus. Childbirth is also called labor. Pregnant humans go into labor roughly nine months after conception.

The first stage of parturition i.e. Dilation starts with the onset of labor. It continues until the cervix is fully dilated. This dilation is divided into two phases; Latent phase: The cervix is 0 to 4 centimeters (cm) dilated and Active phase: The cervix is 4 to 10 cm dilated.The latent phase takes about six hours for a woman who's giving birth for the first time. It takes around five hours for a woman who's given birth previously. For some women, the latent phase may last 8 to 12 hours. During the active phase, it's expected that the cervix will dilate at a rate of about 1 cm per hour for a woman who's giving birth for the first time. For a woman who's previously had a vaginal delivery, the rate is typically about 2 cm per hour (Frothingham, 2018).

The second stage of parturition i.e, Expulsion starts at full dilation and continues until birth. This stage also has two phases: Passive phase: The baby's head moves down through the vagina. Active phase: The mother feels a need to push, or contract the abdominal muscles in time with uterine contractions. The active phase lasts about 45 minutes for a woman who's having her first baby. For women who've had a vaginal delivery, the active phase lasts about 30 minutes. Stage 2 ends with the birth of the baby. At this point, the umbilical cord is clamped, and breastfeeding is often encouraged to help with stage 3 (Frothingham, 2018).

The third stage of parturition i.e. Placental starts after birth and ends with the delivery of the afterbirth (placenta and membranes).If the doctor takes an active role — including gently pulling on the placenta — stage 3 typically takes around five minutes. If the placenta is delivered without assistance, stage 3 can last around 30 minutes (Frothingham, 2018).

The Clitoris consists of a glans, covered by a prepuce and a sub-cutaneous body and it is attached to the under surface of the symphisis by the suspensory ligament. It is well supplied with nerve endings and is extremely sensitive. During coitus, it becomes erect and plays a considerable role in inducing the orgasm in the females.

The Vestibule is the portion between anterior and inner aspects of labia minora and is bounded posteriorly by the vaginal introitus. The outer urinary meatus is immediately posterior to clitoris. The vaginal orifice is situated posteriorly to meatus that is surrounded by the hymen, which is a thin membrane covered on each surface by squamous epithelium. Coitus results in rupture of hymen which may cause a brisk haemorrhage occasionally.

The perineum refers to the area between symphysis of the pubis and coccyx. This is the little flesh between the vagina and the anus present in females. It has a thin layer of subcutaneous fibro-muscular tissue and skin with fewer hair than the rest of the genitalia. The perineum stretches tremendously during childbirth to allow the mother to push the newborn out. This sometimes results in a perineal tear, which can be hard to stitch back up and heal. The goal is to learn to relax the pelvic floor muscles and stretch the vaginal opening (Galan, 2020).

Endocrine Changes

Human pregnancy associated endocrinology involves endocrine and metabolic changes, resulting from various physiological changes at the boundary between mother and the foetus. Along with other hormones, progesterone and oestrogen play an important role. Adequate levels of circulating hormones are of primary importance for normal reproductive function. Successful pregnancy depends on an appropriate maternal immune response to the fetus. (Kumar and Magon, 2012). Profound endocrine changes are essential for the maintenance of pregnancy, normal foetal growth and the postpartum recovery after delivery.

Pituitary Gland

Anatomically, there is a significant enlargement of the pituitary gland during pregnancy. The enlargement of pituitary gland during pregnancy is mainly due to proliferation and an increase in the number of prolactin-producing cells in the anterior lobe, with the proportion of lactotrophs increasing from 1 to 40 percent. This results in elevated prolactin level to 10 to 20 times of the normal non-pregnant value. The increase in prolactin is most likely due to increasing serum oestradiol concentrations during pregnancy. Unless the woman breastfeeds, this increased level returns to normal by 2 weeks of postpartum. The levels of gonadotrophin are reduced by elevated oestrogen and progesterone concentrations, and are undetectable during pregnancy. Serum prolactin levels increase in the first trimester and are 10 times higher at term. It helps in initiation of lactation. However, the high levels of oestrogen and progesterone hormones play an inhibitory role by blocking the binding of prolactin to breast tissues till the birth of the baby (Liu, 2004).

During pregnancy, levels of the basal growth hormone and anti-diuretic hormone remain the same. Owing to negative feedback from elevated levels of oestrogen, progesterone and inhibin, levels of follicle-stimulating hormone (FSH) and luteinising hormone (LH) are undetectable during pregnancy (Prager and Braunstein, 1995). Pituitary growth hormone production is decreased but serum growth hormone levels are increased due to growth hormone production from the placenta (Yanamandra and Chandraharan, 2012).

The posterior pituitary produces oxytocin and Arginine VasoPressin (AVP). Oxytocin levels increase in pregnancy and peak at term. During pregnancy, the uterine contractions is stimulated by this hormone but, until near term, high levels of progesterone secretion prevent contractions of the uterus. After birth, in response to the infants sucking of the breasts of the mother, it also stimulates the let-down or milk-ejection reflex. Anti-diuretic hormone (ADH) levels remain unchanged but the reduction in sodium concentration during pregnancy causes osmolarity to decrease. Then, osmoreceptors for the release and thirst of Anti-Diuretic Hormone (ADH) are reset (Linheimer et al, 1991).

Human Chorionic Gonadotropin (hCG), also referred to as human placental lactogen that is produced by the placenta. This hormone is suggested to act as growth hormone which contributes to the development of breasts. It also helps to reduce maternal glucose metabolism and increase the amount of fatty acids to be used for various metabolic needs (Liu, 2004).

Thyroid Gland

There is increased synthesis of Thyroxine Binding Globulin (TBG) by the liver in pregnancy. This increase of Thyroxine Binding Globulin (TBG) leads to a compensatory rise in serum concentrations of total T3 and T4. Nevertheless, the amounts of thyroid hormones, which circulate freely, remain unchanged. Due to depletion, there is an iodine deficiency caused by the increased glomerular filtration and reduced absorption of the renal tubular. From the second trimester, active transport of iodine to the foeto-placental unit and fetal thyroid function further deplete the maternal iodide supply (Verberg et al, 2005).

Thyroid hormones can also be involved in developing signs of nausea, as a clear correlation has been identified between nausea and irregular thyroid function tests. Thyroid-stimulating hormone (TSH) and HCG have identical bio-molecular structures, and thus HCG interacts with TSH, activating the thyroid gland (Castro et al, 1994). As etiological reasons for nausea and vomiting during pregnancy, psychological causes, genetic incompatibility, immunological factors, nutritional deficiencies and Helicobacter pylori infection were suggested (Verberg et al, 2005).

Adrenal Gland

The serum levels of deoxycorticosterone, corticosteroid-binding globulin (CBG), adreno-corticotropic hormone (ACTH), cortisol and free cortisol often increase throughout pregnancy. Such changes cause a physiological hypercortisolism and can be clinically expressed by striae, facial proliferation, increased blood pressure or decreased glucose tolerance (Gordon, 2012).

Total Cortisol levels rise at the end of the first trimester and at the end of pregnancy, they are three times higher than non-pregnant. In late pregnancy, hypercortisolism is also the outcome of the placenta development of Corticotropin-releasing hormone, which is one of the causes for the initiation of labor. The diurnal fluctuations in the levels of Adreno-Corticotropic Hormone (ACTH) and Cortisol are maintained. The response to exogenous gluco-corticoids in the hypothalamic – pituitary axis is blunted during pregnancy (Gordon, 2012).

During pregnancy, the concentration of plasma CBG (Corticosteroid Binding Globulin) increases. Both free and bound cortisol levels also rise and serum and urinary-free levels of cortisol triple over the full term. In non-pregnant women, the Adreno-Cortico-Tropic Hormone (ACTH) regulating steroid secretion from the adrenal cortex, remains within the normal range.

Physiological Adaptations of Reproductive System

Maternal physiological adaptations during pregnancy are attributed to the hormones of pregnancy and the mechanical pressure exerted by the growing uterus and other related tissues. These adaptations promote normal physiological functioning of the mother, meet the metabolic demands of pregnancy and provide a nurturing environment for the growth and development of the foetus. Though pregnancy is a normal physiological process but complications may occur.

Changes in the Uterus

In the female reproductive system, the uterus, also called the womb, is the hollow organ that carries the foetus during pregnancy. The uterus performs a variety of functions and plays an important role in fertility and childbearing. This organ undergoes change in shape as muscles tighten and relax to allow the carrying of a foetus. The uterus grows during pregnancy, and the muscles get stretched and thinner, like a balloon. The human body would not tolerate the rapid growth of a foetus without this ability of the uterus to expand (Whitlock, 2019).

There are three strata of the uterus. Perimetrium is the external tissue layer which line the outside of the uterus. The Myometrium, the middle layer of the uterus, consists primarily of a smooth muscle. The Endometrium is the innermost layer of the uterus that is the layer that builds up over the course of a month and sheds every month, if there is no pregnancy. The menstrual period is that shedding of the uterus lining. When pregnant, the endometrium provides the fertilized egg with the required nutrients and eventually nurtures the placenta (Whitlock, 2019).

Growth of the uterus is stimulated by the hormones of pregnancy, oestrogen and progesterone which are the chief pregnancy hormones. The hormone Oestrogen promotes the genital, uterine and breast enlargement and increases the vascularity, thus causing vasodilatation. This hormone also causes the pelvic ligaments and joints to relax. It also alters the nutrient metabolism by interfering with the metabolism of folic acid, thereby raising the level of total protein in the body and promoting the retention of sodium and water by the kidney tubules. The rapid increase in oestrogen levels during the first trimester may cause some of the nausea associated with pregnancy. Oestrogen may decrease the secretion of hydrochloric acid and pepsin which is responsible of digestive problems such as nausea. During one pregnancy, a woman will produce more oestrogen than during her entire life, if she is not pregnant. The increase in oestrogen during pregnancy allows the uterus and placenta to improve the vascularization (blood vessel formation), transfer various needed nutrients and support the baby development. Additionally, it is thought that oestrogen plays an important role in helping the foetus for development and maturation. during pregnancy, levels of oestrogen levels increase gradually and reach peak level in the third trimester (Wilson, 2017).

Progesterone causes fat to deposit in the sub-cutaneous tissues over the maternal abdomen, back and upper thighs which serve as an energy reserve for both pregnancy and lactation. The levels of progesterone during pregnancy are also extraordinarily high. Progesterone changes cause ligaments and joints to be lax or loosened throughout the body. Additionally, high progesterone levels cause internal structures, such as the ureters, to increase in size. Maternal bladder connects the ureters to the kidneys. Progesterone again plays an important role in transforming the uterus in its non-pregnant state from the size of a small pear to a fully developed uterus that can accommodate a full-term baby. Progesterone is essential for maintaining pregnancy by relaxing smooth muscles, resulting in decreased uterine contractibility and prevention of miscarriage (Wilson, 2017).

As uterus enlarges, it also changes in its shape and position. At the time of conception, it is like an upside-down pear. During second trimester, it becomes spherical and globular with more elastic and strong muscular walls. Later, it becomes larger and ovoid and rises out of the pelvis into the abdominal cavity. Towards the end, the fundal height drops as the foetus begins to descend and engage in the pelvis.

After conception, the uterus grows to the size of a hen's egg by 7 weeks of gestation, to the size of an orange by 10 weeks of gestation and to the size of a grape fruit by 12 weeks of gestation. After the first trimester, the growth of uterus occurs due to mechanical pressure exerted by the growing foetus. The combination of a weakening of pelvic floor and increased weight places pressure on the pelvis can cause vaginal pressure during the second and third trimesters. In the second trimester, the extra weight of pregnancy often gets more noticeable. The uterus is increasingly putting pressure on the lower body with the progressing pregnancy. With the weakening of pelvic floor, this pressure may cause fullness feeling in the vagina or the generalized hip and pelvic pain and pressure. This pelvic pressure can be an early sign of labor for some women in the later stages of pregnancy (Ernst, 2020).

The uterus normally rotates to the right side as it elevates most probably because of the presence of colon on the left side. Eventually, the growing uterus touches the anterior abdominal wall pushing the intestine to either side of the abdomen. In this position, the uterine fundus presses the urinary bladder, thus increasing the frequency of urination among pregnant women.

After 16 weeks of gestation, the uterine contractions, called **Braxton Hicks Sign**, occur intermittently to facilitate uterine blood flow through placenta and promote the supply of oxygen to the growing foetus. Though irregular and painless in the beginning, these contractions become more definite after 28 weeks of gestation. The uterine muscle, also called the myometrium, consists of individual muscle cells, all of which work together. Those independent cells, called myocytes, contract and flex in isolation during the early days of pregnancy. Sometimes, they join their neighbor myocyte next to it, in an attempt and sometimes they collaborate in small clusters of muscles. At this point, at times the contractions are uncoordinated, isolated and less frequent. This contraction frequency picks up later during pregnancy but is still uncoordinated across the uterus. These pesky Braxton Hicks contractions, on a physiological level, are like small muscle twitches, just sporadic moments of uterine muscle flexing. They often get felt at one spot or as intermittent tightening which is quite different from labor contractions (Dickens, 2020).

As the uterus increases in size, blood flow to the uterus also increases rapidly. Although uterine blood flow increases twenty-fold, the foeto-placental unit grows more rapidly. These are achieved through establishing multiple communication systems in which a large array of substances produced by the foeto-placental unit reach and modulate specific maternal target organs and/or systems. Myometrium is a fundamental reproductive tissue involved in the maintenance of pregnancy as well as the onset and progression of labour and is a potential target organ for such a communication system. Appropriate regulation of myometrial function is a key condition that will be required for pregnancy to develop physiologically till reaching the full term and labor begins. It is suggested through the emerging experimental and clinical evidence that an extremely complex bio-molecular feto-placental communication system exists with the myometrium and is actively operational in the control of myometrial contractility during pregnancy as well as parturition by producing a continuously rising number of substances with the actions of endocrine, paracrine, and immune-regulations (Ticconi, 2006).

About one-sixth of the total maternal blood volume lies in the uterine vascular system in a normal pregnancy. The rate of blood flow averages 500 ml/min through the uterus and the supply of oxygen to the gravid uterus rises to meet the requirements of the growing foetus. However, the uterine blood flow may be decreased due to a low maternal arterial pressure, contractions of the uterus and the maternal supine position. Oestrogen stimulation may increase the uterine blood flow. To measure the uterine blood flow velocity in high risk pregnancies because of the conditions associated with decreased placental perfusions, hypertension, diabetes mellitus, intra-uterine growth retardation and multiple gestation, Doppler ultrasound examination may be used (Harman, 2004).

During childbirth, the uterus contracts to help push the fetus from the body (Gossman et al, 2019). These contractions with a series of muscle movements squeeze the foetus out of the uterus and into the vagina. The uterus continues to contract after the baby is born, which helps the organ to revert to its normal size. It also helps to stop bleeding which takes place during delivery in the uterus (Whitlock, 2019).

Cervical Changes

At six weeks of gestation, softening of the cervical tip is called **Goodell Sign.** It is caused by an increased vascularity, slight hypertrophy and hyperplasia of the muscle and its collagen rich connective tissue which becomes loose, edematous, highly elastic and increased in volume. A velvety appearance of the cervix caused by the secretion of the glands is characteristic sign of pregnancy. Friability is increased and may cause slight bleeding after coitus or after vaginal examination. Careful examination of all pregnant women is important because about 3 percent of all cervical cancers are diagnosed during pregnancy (Berman, DiSaia and Tiwari, 2004).

Leucorrhea is a white or grey mucoid discharge with a faint musty odour which occurs in response to cervical stimulation by oestogen and progesterone. The effect of progesterone does not let ferning occur in the dried cervical mucous smear as in a smear of amniotic fluid. Instead, a cellular crystallizing pattern is formed in the dried mucous (Gibbs, Sweet and Duff, 2004).

During ovulation, mucus is produced to assist sperm pass through the cervix and give a an ideal environment before the fertilization of an egg. Once fertilization occurs, the mucus changes to seal the cervix, called the mucus plug to protect the fetus from infection (Ritchfield et al, 2013). The mucus plug is formed from secretions of cervical glands and has a thick, gelatinous consistency (Ritchfield et al, 2013).

The mucous fills the endocervical canal, resulting in the formation of mucous plug, **Operculum**, which acts as a barrier against bacterial invasion during pregnancy. Moreover, the acidic vaginal secretion (pH ranging 3.5 to 6.0) caused by the increased production of lactic acid by *Lactobacillus acidophilus* action on glycogen in the vaginal epithelium, results from the increased secretion of oestrogen during pregnancy (Cunningham et al, 2005). Though this acidic medium provides protection against some organisms but it makes the pregnant women more vulnerable to other infections, especially the yeast infection as the glycogen rich environment is susceptible to infection by *Candida albicans* (Gibbs, Sweet and Duff, 2004). Lacerations of cervix occur during the childbirth. After child birth, the cervix becomes more oval in the horizontal plane, with or without lacerations.

When the fertilized egg implants into the wall of the uterus, the plug begins to form. As this occurs, as mucosal cells begin to pump mucus into the cavity until no gaps are left, the cervix softens and swells. The mucus thickens and continuously gets secreted throughout pregnancy, prompted by the hormone progesterone, so that the plug always stays fresh. Antibodies are present inside this thick, sticky fluid which provides protection to the growing foetus from many bacteria, viruses and other agents that cause disease. The rupture of the capillaries may also cause streaks of red or pink, which is why the loss of the mucus plug is sometimes referred to as the "bloody show." The passing of the plug is an indication of the sign that labor is nearing, regardless of the pregnancy stage. Therefore, the mucus plug passing during early pregnancy is the sign of impending preterm birth (Weiss, 2020).

Changes in the Vagina and Vulva

The pregnancy hormones make the vagina ready to stretch during childbirth. This happens when the vaginal mucosa thickens, the connective tissues loosens, the smooth muscles hypertrophy and the vaginal vault lengthens. The vaginal mucosa and the cervix turn violet bluish as a result of increased vascularity. The deepened colour, known as **Chadwick Sign**, is noticed at 8 weeks of gestation (Monga and Sanborn, 2004).

Changes in Breasts

Among the earliest signs of pregnancy are changes in the breast. This is because of the progesterone hormone. Additionally, the dark skin areas around the nipples (the areolas) start swelling. This is followed by the breasts themselves swelling fast. Most pregnant women feel soreness on the sides of their breasts, and tingling or soreness in their nipples. This is because the milk duct system is growing and many more lobules are formed.

As a result of increased levels of oestrogen and progestrone in pregnant women, fullness and heaviness of breasts, increased sensitivity and tingling sensation occurs during early pregnancy. Nipples and areolae become more pigmented, secondary pink areolae develop beyond the primary areolae and erectile the nipples. In the primary areolae, hypertrophy of sebaceous glands can be seen around the nipples which have a protective role in keeping the nipples lubricated for breastfeeding. The blood vessels beneath the skin dilate due to rich supply of blood, showing an intertwining blue network of blood vessels beneath the surface of the skin.

By the fifth or sixth month of pregnancy, the breasts can produce milk to the full. As in puberty, the growth of ducts is controlled by estrogen, and that of glandular buds are controlled by progesterone. In milk production many other hormones also play vital roles. These include follicle-stimulating hormone (FSH), luteinizing hormone (LH), prolactin, oxytocin and placental lactogen (HPL) in humans (Hopkins, 2020).

During the second and the third trimester, progressive enlargement of breasts takes place as a result of growth of mammary glands. The high levels of luteal and placental hormones promote proliferation of lactiferous ducts and lobule-alvoelar tissues. Glandular tissues replace connective tissues and tissues become softer and looser. Though the mammary glands are fully developed by mid pregnancy but lactation is inhibited by a decrease in oestrogen level till the birth of the child. A clear viscous secretion, called pre-colostrum, is seen in the acini cells by the third month of gestation. A creamy white to yellow fluid, called Colostrum, is secreted as early as 16 weeks of gestation (Lawrence and Lawrence, 2004).

Gastrointestinal Tract Changes

As pregnancy progresses, there also occur mechanical changes in the alimentary tract that are triggered by the growing uterus. The stomach is rising upwards gradually, leading to an altered axis and increased intra-gastric pressure. The tone of the oesophageal sphincter is also reduced, and these factors can predispose to reflux symptoms leading to nausea and vomiting commonly experienced by pregnant women (Koch, 2002).

Changes in pregnancy hormones, oestrogen and progesterone levels also affect the structural alterations in the gastrointestinal tract. These changes include abnormalities in gastric neural activity and smooth functioning of the muscle, thus leading to gastic dysrhythmia or gastroparesis. In pregnant women with pre-existing gastrointestinal diseases such as gastro-esophageal reflux disease, diabetic gastroparesis, gastric bypass surgery or inflammatory bowel diseases, such changes are pronounced (Clark et al, 2012).

Nausea and vomiting are very common complaints in pregnancy, affecting 50 to 90 percent of pregnancies. This could be an adaptive function of pregnancy that aims to prevent pregnant women from eating potentially teratogenic items such as strong tasting fruits and vegetables. The exact underlying mechanism is not clear, but it could include pregnancy-associated hormones such as human Chorionic Gonadotropin (hCG), estrogen and progesterone in its etiology. The human hormone Chorionic Gonadotropin(hCG) level peaks at the end of the first trimester when the trophoblast most actively releases human Chorionic Gonadotropin (hCG), which is associated with the symptoms of nausea. Nausea is also more common in pregnancies with elevated human chorionic gonadotropin (hCG) levels, such as twin pregnancies (American College of Obstetrics and Gynecology (ACOG) Practice Bulletin, 2004).

Nevertheless, the nausea symptoms usually resolve by week 20 of gestation but about 10 to 20 percent of pregnant women experience symptoms after week 20 and some until the end of pregnancy. In most cases, minor dietary changes and electrolyte balance observations are adequate. Around 0.5 to 3 per cent of pregnant women experience hyperemesis gravidum, an extreme and persistent form of nausea and frequent vomiting also leading to dehydration, electrolyte imbalance, ketonuria, weight loss and deficiencies in vitamins or minerals (American College of Obstatrics and Gynecology (ACOG) Practice Bulletin, 2004; Clark et al, 2012). In these cases, intravenous fluid and vitamin substitution is commonly required. Thiamine supplementation is important in order to avoid the development of Wernicke's encephalopathy (Niebyl and Goodwin, 2002).

Cardiovascular Changes

Anatomically, with lateral displacement of the left border, the heart is gradually pushed upwards and rotated forward. The sounds of the heart are louder and the first sound splits. In 88 per cent of the cases, a loud, widely split first sound occurs during pregnancy due to early closure of the mitral valve. No change occurs in the second sound, other than poor movement in late pregnancy of the two elements. In 84 per cent of cases, a loud third sound occurs. In 16 per cent of cases, an occasional fourth sound also occurs. Ninety-two percent of the patients revealed the signs of a systolic murmur of the ejection type. An "early" diastolic murmur occurs in 9 cases; this murmur is on account of flow murmur from the atrio-ventricular valve. A systolic ejection murmur is common and is caused by secondary turbulence to an increased blood flow through normal heart valves. Occasionally, a diastolic murmur is heard (Cutforth & MacDonald 1966).

The primary physiological adaptation during pregnancy is probably the peripheral vasodilatation. This results in a 25 to 30 percent reduction in systemic vascular resistance and cardiac output rises by around 40 percent to compensate for this during pregnancy. This is done mostly through an improvement in the number of strokes but also to a lesser degree through an increase in heart rate. The highest cardiac output is estimated at 20 to 28 weeks gestational time. An increase in stroke volume is possible due to the early increase in ventricular wall muscle mass and end-diastolic volume (Yanamandra and Chandraharan, 2012).

Changes in the cardiovascular system during pregnancy are significant and start as early as eight weeks of gestation during pregnancy, cardiac production has already been raised by 20 percent. From initial pregnancy, the total volume of blood is steadily increasing to a maximum of 35-45 percent above the non-pregnant level at 32 weeks of gestation. The volume of plasma increases by 40 percent while the mass of red cells increases by 20 percent, thus leading to haemodilution i.e. physiological anaemia (Mowafi, 2019).

Cardiac output is increased as a result of increased heart rate, reduced systemic vascular resistance and increased stroke. This value increases to 25 percent by the end of the second trimester but there is no volume. Heart rate is increased above the non-pregnant values by 15 percent at the end of the first trimester further change in the heart rate during the third trimester. Stroke volume is raised by about 20 percent at 8 weeks of gestation and up to 30 percent by the concluding of the second trimester and then is constant until full term of pregnancy (Yanamandra and Chandraharan, 2012).

A relationship exists between the raised levels of estrogen and progesterone and vasodilatation (Walters, 1969) and, of course, both levels rise significantly during pregnancies. Relaxin is a peptide hormone which is produced by the circulating corpus luteum during pregnancy. It is detectable in ovulatory cycle luteal phase. When conception occurs, serum concentrations peak at the end of the first trimester and fall throughout pregnancy to an intermediate value (Conrad, 2011). This hormone has been shown to have an endothelium-dependent vasodilatory function during pregnancy which can affect the small vessels of arterial resistance (Fisher et al, 2002).

The heart is physiologically dilated and myocardial contractibility is increased. Although stroke volume declines towards the full term of pregnancy but the maternal heart rate changes (10 to 20 bpm) are preserved, thereby maintaining increased cardiac output. Blood pressure drops in the first and second trimesters but during the third trimester of pregnancy, it rises to non-pregnant stage.

A further increase in cardiac output (15 percent in the first stage and 50 percent in the second) is correlated with the delivery. Uterine contractions result in an auto-transfusion of 300 to 500 ml of blood back into the bloodstream and the heart rate and blood pressure is elevated further in sympathetic response to pain and anxiety. Between the contractions, the cardiac output is increased but more so during the contractions.

After birth, the cardiac output instantly increases due to relief of the inferior vena cava obstruction and uterine contraction that empties blood into the systemic circulation. There is an increase in cardiac output by 60 to 80 percent, followed by a rapid decrease in pre-labor value within approximately one hour of supply. There is an improvement in venous return and further stroke volume by fluid transfer from the extra vascular space.

Therefore, some pregnant women with cardio-vascular dysfunction are mostly at risk of pulmonary oedema during the second labor stage and immediate postpartum period. Two weeks after delivery, cardiac output has almost returned to normal (pre-pregnancy value), though some pathological changes (e.g. pre-eclampsia hypertension) may take much longer to overcome (Pillay, 2016).

Those unfamiliar with pregnancy physiological adaptations may misinterpret the above physiological changes as pathological changes on cardiovascular examination. These changes may include a bounding or collapsing pulse, and a systolic murmur of ejection, present in over 90 percent of pregnant women. The murmur can be loud and audible throughout the precordium, with the first loud heart sound and possibly sometimes a third heart sound also. Also, ectopic beats and peripheral oedema may be present (Pillay, 2016).

Respiratory Changes

The subjective feeling of breathlessness without hypoxia may occur during pregnancy as a result of physiological adaptation and is most common during third trimester. However, it may start any time during gestation. Moreover, breathlessness is present at rest and may increase during mild activity.

Anatomically, nasal and pharyngeal mucosa and larynx capillary engorgement starts as early as in the first trimester. This can explain why many pregnant women complain of nasal breathing problems, experience more episodes of epistaxis and experience changes in voice. The thoracic cage increases in circumference by 5 to 7 cm because of the increase in both the antero-posterior and transverse diameters from flaring of the ribs. During pregnancy, the diaphragm level rises by about 4 cm early, even before it is under mechanical pressure from the enlarged uterus. This accounts for the decline in the residual volume since at the forced expiration, the lungs would be compressed relatively (Yanamandra and Chandraharan, 2012).

During late pregnancy, the decreased functional residual capacity may result due to diaphragmatic elevation. Due to an increased tidal volume, inspiratory reserve volume is decreased early during pregnancy but rises in the third trimester as a result of reduced functional residual capacity. However, during pregnancy, the peak expiratory flow rate (PEFR) and the forced expiratory volume in one second (FEV1) are not affected (Mowafi, 2019).

There is a significant increase in oxygen demand during normal pregnancy. This is due to 15 percent increase in the metabolic rate and 20 percent increased oxygen consumption. In minute ventilation, there is a rise of 40 to 50 per cent on account of an increase in tidal volume rather than in respiratory rate. This maternal hyperventilation results in an increase in arterial pO2 and a fall in arterial pCO2, with a compensatory reduction of 18 to 22 mmol / l in the serum bicarbonate. Consequently, a mild, fully compensated respiratory alkalosis is normal in pregnancy (arterial pH 7.44).

Renal Changes

During pregnancy, anatomical renal changes include an improvement in the length of the kidney by around 1 cm. Renal calyces, pelvis, and the ureters are all markedly dilated. A rise of around 50 per cent in the Glomerular Filtration Rate (GFR) reaches the maximum level at the end of the first trimester and remains at this elevated level until at least 36th week of gestation. Twenty-four-hour creatinine clearance increases by 25 percent at 4 weeks of gestation after the last menstrual period and by 45 percent at 9 weeks of gestation. During the third trimester, a consistent and significant decrease towards non-pregnant value occurs preceding the delivery (Yanamandra and Chandraharan, 2012).

As a consequence of renal vasodilatation, Renal Plasma Flow (RPF) and Glomerular Filtration Rate (GFR) both increase as compared to the non-pregnant levels by 40 to 65 percent and 50 to 85 percent respectively. In addition, the increase in plasma volume causes decreased osmotic pressure in the glomeruli, with a subsequent rise in Glomerular Filtration Rate (Cheung and Lafayette, 2013).

Moreover, in both the renal afferent and efferent arterioles, vascular resistance decreases and therefore, despite the massive rise in renal plasma flow, glomerular hydrostatic pressure remains stable, thereby preventing the development of glomerular hypertension. As the Glomerular Filtration Rate (GFR) increases, the concentrations of both serum creatinine and urea drops to mean respective values of about 44.2 μmol / l and 3.2 mmol / l (Cheung and Lafayette, 2013).

The increased renal blood flow leads to an increase in renal size of 1 to 1.5 cm, hit the maximum size by the middle of pregnancy. Due to mechanical compressive pressures on the ureters, the kidneys, pelvis and calyceum system dilate. Such anatomical changes are mediated by progesterone, which decreases the ureteral tone, peristalsis and contraction pressure (Cheung and Lafayette, 2013).

An increase in kidney vasculature, interstitial volume and dead space in the urine result in an increase in renal size. The ureters, renal pelvis and calyces are also dilated, leading to physiological hydronephrosis in over 80 percent of pregnant women (Rasmussen and Nielsen, 1988). Due to the anatomical conditions of the right ureter, there is often a right-sided predominance of hydronephrosis, which crosses the iliac and ovarian vessels at an angle before reaching the pelvis. In dilated collection system, urinary stasis predisposes pregnant women with asymptomatic bacteriuria to pyelonephritis (Rasmussen and Nielsen, 1988).

The tubular treatment of waste and nutrients often requires physiological alterations. Like in the non-pregnant state, glucose in the glomerulus is freely filtered. For variable excretion, the reabsorption of glucose in the proximal tubule and the collecting tubule is less successful during pregnancy. About 90 per cent of pregnant women with normal levels of blood glucose excrete 1 to 10 gm of glucose per day (Diabetes Quebec, 2020).

As both Glomerular Filtration Rate (GFR) and Glomerular Capillary Permeability (GCP) to albumin increase, protein fractional excretion can increase to 300 mg per day and protein excretion can rise as well. The overall concentration of protein in urine does not rise above the normal upper limit for normal pregnancies. Excretion of uric acid also increases with increased Glomerular Filtration Rate (GFR) and/or decreased tubular reabsorption (Cheung and Lafayette, 2013).

Skeletal Changes

The effect of pregnancy on maternal bone loss is controversial. Although there is an association of pregnancy and lactation with reversible bone loss, research studies do not indicate a correlation between parity and osteoporosis in later life (Dorr et al, 1989).

To support the contributing effect of pregnancy later in life and lactation on osteoporosis, there are some hypotheses. High demand of calcium and low estrogenic state during pregnancy and lactation support those hypotheses. The issue has been investigated in numerous studies but there is no consensus on the contributing effect of pregnancy and lactation on osteoporosis. Thus, pregnancy may result in bone loss but if lactation is followed, it will have a protective effect on bone density, though the duration of lactation and parity may modulate its effect (Salari and Abdollahi, 2014).

In the first trimester, bone turnover is low and rises in the third trimester as the calcium needs of foetus increase. The calcium source in the third trimester is skeletal calcium which has been already deposited (Woodrow et al, 2006).

A study of bone biopsies in pregnancy has shown a change in the micro-architectural pattern of bone during pregnancy but not overall bone mass (Woodrow et al, 2006). The changes reflect the need for the maternal skeleton to be resistant to bending forces and biochemical stresses needed to carry the growing foetus.

Metabolic Changes

During pregnancy, the maternal metabolism changes significantly. Early gestation can be seen in the mother as an anabolic state with a rise in maternal fat stores and small decline in the sensitivity to insulin. Thus nutrients are stored in early pregnancy to meet the late gestation and lactation feto-placental and maternal demands. On the contrary, late pregnancy is characterized as a catabolic state with reduced sensitivity to insulin i.e. an increased resistance to insulin. An increase in insulin resistance results in increased concentrations of maternal glucose and free fatty acid, thus enabling greater availability of substrates for foetal growth (Lain and Catalano, 2007).

Glucose Metabolism

Pregnancy is a diabetogenic state and glucose metabolism adaptations allow the thrusting of glucose to promote the development of the foetus while maintaining the adequate levels of maternal nutrition (Angueira et al, 2015). Insulin-secreting pancreatic beta-cells undergo hyperplasia, resulting in increased insulin secretion and increased insulin sensitivity in early pregnancy followed by progressive insulin resistance (Butte, 2000).

Pregnancy is associated with an insulin-resistant condition, similar to that of type II diabetes. In a normal pregnancy, maternal tissues become increasingly insensitive to insulin. With advancing gestation, both in women with normal glucose tolerance and in women with gestational diabetes, a decline in insulin sensitivity of 50 to 60 per cent are seen. In women with normal glucose tolerance, a sufficient increase in insulin production from pancreatic beta cells overcomes the changes in insulin sensitivity. However, endogenous insulin secretion is insufficient during pregnancy in women with diabetes. Rising levels of oestrogen and progesterone, which contribute to pancreatic beta-cell hypertrophy and insulin excretion, alter the metabolism of maternal carbohydrates early in pregnancy. Other hormones including human placental lactogen, prolactin, cortisol, oestrogen and progesterone secretion cause insulin resistance. In pregnant women, these hormones are found to be significantly higher (Catalano, 2014).

In the second trimester, maternal insulin resistance begins and reaches its peak in the third trimester. This results from increased diabetes hormone secretion such as human placental lactogen, growth hormone, progesterone, cortisol, and prolactin, thereby causing insulin sensitivity to decrease in peripheral tissues, such as adipocytes and skeletal muscles, by interfering with insulin receptor signaling (Newbern and Freemark, 2011). The effect of the placental hormones on insulin sensitivity is made evident during postpartum when there is a sudden decrease in insulin resistance (Mazaki-Tovi et al, 2011).

Throughout pregnancy, insulin levels are raised in the both fasting and postprandial states. Nevertheless, fastening glucose levels are reduced due to increased accumulation of tissue glycogen, increased use of peripheral glucose, decreased production of glucose by the liver and absorption of glucose by the foetus (Brizzi et al, 1999).

Lipolysis results from the insulin resistance and relative hypoglycaemia, thereby enabling the pregnant mother to use fat preferentially for fuel, thus maintaining the available foetal glucose and amino acids and reducing the catabolism of proteins. The placenta allows glucose, amino acids, and ketones to be passed to the foetus but is impermeable to large molecules of lipids. If a woman has compromised her endocrine pancreatic function and she is not able to overcome the pregnancy-related insulin resistance, it results in the development of gestational diabetes.

Lipid Metabolism

During pregnancy, total serum cholesterol and triglyceride levels rise. The rise in triglyceride level is mainly due to its increased synthesis in the liver and decrease in lipoprotein lipase activity, leading to a decreased adipose tissue catabolism. The cholesterol level in low-density lipoprotein (LDL) also rises and exceeds 50 per cent at the full term. There is an increase in the high-density lipoprotein level in the first half of pregnancy which decreases in the third trimester. However, its concentration is higher by 15 percent as compared to the level in non-pregnant state.

The needs of the developing foetus are accommodated by the changes in lipid metabolism. Increased levels of triglycerides cater to the energy needs of pregnant mother while the foetus is also spared glucose. For placental steroidogenesis, the increase in LDL cholesterol is significant.

Protein Metabolism

During pregnancy, pregnant women require an elevated level of protein intake. Amino acids are constantly transferred through the placenta to meet the growing foetus ' needs. Protein catabolism is decreased during pregnancy, as fat stores are used to meet the need of energy metabolism.

CONCLUSION

In the absence of pregnancy, the levels of oestrogen and progesterone gradually decline and the decline in the level of these hormones results in menstruation. A decline in the level of these hormones also initiates a fresh positive feedback mechanism and triggers gonadotropin release from the hypothalamus. This is how menstrual cycle is regulated. Because of the anatomical and physiological changes occurring during pregnancy, understanding the investigations in the light of the changed values is necessary. Specific ranges of reference for pregnancy should be used in clinical decision making.

REFERENCES

American College of Obstetrics and Gynaecology (ACOG) Practice Bulletin. (2004). Nausea and vomiting of pregnancy. *Obstetrics and Gynecology, 103*(4), 803–814. doi:10.1097/00006250-200404000-00045 PMID:15051578

Angueira, A. R., Ludvik, A. E., Reddy, T. E., Wicksteed, B., Lowe, W. L. Jr, & Layden, B. T. (2015). New insights into gestational glucose metabolism: Lessons learned from 21st century approaches. *Diabetes, 64*(2), 327–334. doi:10.2337/db14-0877 PMID:25614666

Berman, M., DiSaia, P., & Tiwari, K. (2004). Pelvic Malignancies, Gestational Trophoplastic Neoplasia and Non- Pelvic Malignancies. In Maternal Fetal Medicines: Principles and Practice (5th ed.). Philadelphia, Saunders.

Boutot, M. (2019). *How pregnancy actually happens? Concepts of Biology - 1st Canadian Edition by Charles Molnar and Jane Gair (2019).* Retrieved from https://helloclue.com/articles/sex/conception-pregnancy-fertilization-explained

Brizzi, Tonolo, G., Esposito, F., Puddu, L., Dessole, S., Maioli, M., & Milia, S. (1999). Lipoprotein metabolism during normal pregnancy. *American Journal of Obstetrics and Gynecology, 81*(2), 430–434. doi:10.1016/S0002-9378(99)70574-0 PMID:10454696

Butte, N. F. (2000). Carbohydrate and lipid metabolism in pregnancy: Normal compared with gestational diabetes mellitus. *The American Journal of Clinical Nutrition*, *71*(5), 125S. doi:10.1093/ajcn/71.5.1256s PMID:10799399

Castro, L. C., Hobel, C. J., & Gornbein, J. (1994). Plasma levels of atrial natriuretic peptide in normal and hypertensive pregnancies: A meta-analysis. *American Journal of Obstetrics and Gynecology*, *171*(6), 1642–1651. doi:10.1016/0002-9378(94)90416-2 PMID:7802082

Catalano, P. M. (2014). Trying to understand gestational diabetes. *Diabetic Medicine*, *31*(3), 273–281. doi:10.1111/dme.12381 PMID:24341419

Cheung, K. L., & Lafayette, R. A. (2013). Renal physiology of pregnancy. *Advances in Chronic Kidney Disease*, *20*(3), 209–214. doi:10.1053/j.ackd.2013.01.012 PMID:23928384

Clark, S. M., Costantine, M. M., & Hankins, G. F. (2012). Review of NVP and HG and early pharmacotherapeutic intervention. *Obstetrics and Gynecology International*, *2012*, 252676. doi:10.1155/2012/252676 PMID:22190950

Conrad, K. P. (2011). Emerging role of relaxin in the maternal adaptations to normal pregnancy: Implications for preeclampsia. *Seminars in Nephrology*, *31*(1), 15–32. doi:10.1016/j.semnephrol.2010.10.003 PMID:21266262

Cunningham, F., Leveno, K., Bloom, S., Hauth, J., Gilstrap, L., & Wenstrom, K. (2005). Williams Obstetrics (22nd ed.). McGraw-Hill.

Cutforth, R., & MacDonald, C. B. (1966). Heart sounds and murmurs in pregnancy. *American Heart Journal*, *71*(6), 741–747. doi:10.1016/0002-8703(66)90594-1 PMID:5945138

Diabetes Quebe. (2020). *Diabetes in Pregnancy*. Retrieved from https://www.diabete.qc.ca/en/understand-diabetes/all-about-diabetes/types-of-diabetes/diabetes-in-pregnancy/

Dickens, M. (2020). *The Physiological Difference Between Braxton Hicks and Labor Contractions*. Retrieved from https://bloomlife.com/preg-u/difference-between-braxton-hicks-and-labor-contractions/

Dorr, H. G., Heller, A., Versmold, H. T., Sippell, W. G., Herrmann, M., Bidlingmaier, F., & Knorr, D. (1989). Longitudinal study of progestins, mineralocorticoids and glucocorticoids throughout human pregnancy. *The Journal of Clinical Endocrinology and Metabolism*, *68*(5), 863–868. doi:10.1210/jcem-68-5-863 PMID:2715289

Ernst, H. (2020). *Is having vaginal pressure during pregnancy normal?* Retrieved from https://www.medicalnewstoday.com/articles/322304

Fathalla, M.F. (1999). *Health and Being a Woman.* Figo.org/sites/default/files/uploads/PublicationsandResourcesFathallahfiles/A/4%20Health%20and%20being%20a%20woman.pdf.

Fisher, C., MacLean, M., Morecroft, I., Seed, A., Johnston, F., Hillier, C., & McMurray, J. (2002). Is the pregnancy hormone relaxin also a vasodilator peptide secreted by the heart? *Circulation, 106*(3), 292–295. doi:10.1161/01.CIR.0000025630.05387.45 PMID:12119241

Frothigham, S. (2018). *Three stages of Parturition (Childbirth).* Retrieved from https://www.healthline.com/health/parturition

Galan, N. (2020). *The Importance of the Perineum in Childbirth.* Retrieved from https://www.verywellhealth.com/the-perineum-2616422

Gibbs, R., Sweet, R., & Duff, W. (2004). Maternal and Fetal Infectious Disorders. In R. Creasry, R. Resnik, & J. Iams (Eds.), Maternal Fetal Medicines: Principles and Practice (5th ed.). Philadelphia, Saunders.

Gordon, M. C. (2012). *Maternal Physiology in Obstetrics: Normal and Problem pregnancies. Elsevier* (6th ed.). Saunders.

Gossman, W., Fagan, S. E., & Sosa-Stanley, J. N. (2019). Anatomy, abdomen and pelvis, uterus. In *Stat Pearls*. Stat Pearls Publishing.

Government of Western Australia, Department of Health. (2019). *Pregnancy and Birth: A Brief Overview of Biology and Physiology.* https://gdhr.wa.gov.au/-/pregnan-1

Harman, C. (2004). Assessment of Fetal Health. In R. Creasry, R. Resnik, & J. Iams (Eds.), Maternal Fetal Medicines: Principles and Practice (5th ed.). Philadelphia, Saunders.

Hill, M. A. (2020). *Embryology Implantation.* Retrieved from https://embryology.med.unsw.edu.au/embryology/index.php/Implantation

Holland, E. & Brew, A. (1998). *Manual of Obstetrics* (16th ed.). Academic Press.

Hopkins, J. (2020). *Normal Breast Development and Changes.* https://www.hopkinsmedicine.org/health/conditions-and-diseases/normal-breast-development-and-changes

Howkins & Bourne. (1999). *Shaw's Textbook of Gynaecology* (12th ed.). B.I. Churchill Livingstone Pvt. Ltd.

Ireland, M. L. (2000). The Effects of Pregnancy on the Musculoskeletal System. *Clinical Orthopaedics and Related Research*, (372): 169–179.

Jones, R. E., & Lopez, K. H. (2006). Human Reproductive Biology. Elsevier.

Kampmann, U., Knorr, S., Fuglsang, J & Ovesen, P. (2019). Determinants of Maternal Insulin Resistance during Pregnancy: An Updated Overview. *Journal of Diabetes Research.*

Koch, K. L. (2002). Gastrointestinal factors in nausea and vomiting of pregnancy. *American Journal of Obstetrics and Gynecology*, *186*(5), S198–S203. doi:10.1067/mob.2002.122598 PMID:12011886

Kumar, P., & Magon, N. (2012). Hormones in Pregnancy. *Nigerian Medical Journal*, *53*(4), 179–183. doi:10.4103/0300-1652.107549 PMID:23661874

Lain, K. Y., & Catalano, P. M. (2007). Metabolic changes in pregnancy. *Clinical Obstetrics and Gynecology*, *50*(4), 938–948. doi:10.1097/GRF.0b013e31815a5494 PMID:17982337

Lawrence, R., & Lawrence, R. (2004). The breast and the physiology of lactation. In R. Creasry, R. Resnik, & J. Iams (Eds.), Maternal Fetal Medicines: Principles and Practice (5th ed.). Philadelphia: Saunders.

Linheimer, M. D., Barron, W. M., & Davison, J. M. (1991). Osmotic and volume control of vasopressin release in pregnancy. *American Journal of Kidney Diseases*, *17*(2), 105–111. doi:10.1016/S0272-6386(12)81112-7 PMID:1992649

Liu, J. (2004). Endocrinology of pregnancy. In R. Creasry, R. Resnik, & J. Iams (Eds.), Maternal Fetal Medicines: Principles and Practice (5th ed.). Philadelphia: Saunders.

Locktich, G. (1997). Clinical biochemistry of pregnancy. *Critical Reviews in Clinical Laboratory Sciences*, *34*, 6. PMID:9055057

Mazaki-Tovi, S., Kanety, H., Pariente, C., Hemi, R., Yissachar, E., Schiff, E., Cohen, O., & Sivan, E. (2011). Insulin sensitivity in late gestational and early postpartum period: The role of circulating maternal adipokines. *Gynecological Endocrinology*, *27*(9), 725–731. doi:10.3109/09513590.2010.500426 PMID:21714696

Monga, M., & Sanborn, M. (2004). Biology and physiology of the reproductive tract and control of myometrial contraction. In R. Creasry, R. Resnik, & J. Iams (Eds.), Maternal Fetal Medicines: Principles and Practice (5th ed.). Philadelphia: Saunders.

Moore, K. L., Persaud, T. V. N., & Torchia, M. G. (2016). *The Developing Human E-Book: Clinically Oriented Embryology*. Elsevier Health Sciences.

Mowafi, D. M. (2019). *Maternal changes due to pregnancy*. Retrieved from https://www.gfmer.ch/Obstetrics_simplified/Maternal_changes_due_to_pregnancy.htm

Newbern, D., & Freemark, M. (2011). Placental hormones and the control of maternal metabolism and fetal growth. *Current Opinion in Endocrinology, Diabetes, and Obesity*, *18*(6), 409–416. doi:10.1097/MED.0b013e32834c800d PMID:21986512

Niebyl, J. R., & Goodwin, J. M. (2002). Overview of nausea and vomiting of pregnancy with an emphasis on vitamins and ginger. *American Journal of Obstetrics and Gynecology*, *186*(5), S253–S255. doi:10.1067/mob.2002.122595 PMID:12011896

Padubidri, V. G., & Daftary, S. N. (1999). *Shaw's Textbook of Gynecology*. Churchill Livingstone Pvt. Ltd.

Panawala, L. (2017). *Difference Between Spermatogenesis and Oogenesis*. Retrieved from file:///C:/Users/hp/Desktop/DifferenceBetweenSpermatogenesisand OogenesisDefinitionCharacteristicsFunction20(6).pdf

Pandit, N. (1991). *Pregnancy: The Complete Childbirth Book*. Rupa & Co., Kolkatta.

Pillay, P. S., Catherine, N. P., Tolppanen, H., & Mebazaa, A. (2016). Physiological changes in pregnancy. *Cardiovascular Journal of Africa*, *27*(2), 89–94. doi:10.5830/CVJA-2016-021 PMID:27213856

Prager, D., & Braunstein, G. (1995). Pituitary disorders during pregnancy. *Endocrinology and Metabolism Clinics of North America*, *24*(1), 1–14. doi:10.1016/S0889-8529(18)30051-3 PMID:7781620

Rasmussen, P. E., & Nielsen, F. R. (1988). Hydronephrosis during pregnancy: A literature survey. *European Journal of Obstetrics, Gynecology, and Reproductive Biology*, *27*(3), 249–259. doi:10.1016/0028-2243(88)90130-X PMID:3280355

Ritchfield, A. S., Yao, G., & Jaishankar, A. (2013). Cervical mucus properties stratify risk for preterm birth. *PLoS One*, *8*(8). doi:10.1371/journal.pone.0069528 PMID:23936335

Salari, P., & Abdollahi, M. (2014). The influence of pregnancy and lactation on maternal bone health: A systematic review. *Journal of Family & Reproductive Health*, *8*(4), 135. PMID:25530765

Stanford Children's Health. (2020). *The First Trimester*. Retrieved from https://www.stanfordchildrens.org/en/topic/default?id=first-trimester-85-P01218

Suarez, S. S., & Pacey, A. A. (2006). Sperm transport in the female reproductive tract. *Human Reproduction Update*, *12*(1), 23–37. doi:10.1093/humupd/dmi047 PMID:16272225

Tan, E. K., & Tan, E. L. (2013). Alterations in physiology and anatomy during pregnancy. *Best Practice & Research. Clinical Obstetrics & Gynaecology*, *27*(6), 791–802. doi:10.1016/j.bpobgyn.2013.08.001 PMID:24012425

Thompson, L. (2019a). *The Ovaries*. Retrieved from https://teachmeanatomy.info/pelvis/female-reproductive-tract/ovaries/

Thompson, L. (2019b). *The Vagina*. Retrieved from https://teachmeanatomy.info/pelvis/female-reproductive-tract/vagina/

Thompson, L. (2020). *The Cervix*. Retrieved from https://teachmeanatomy.info/pelvis/female-reproductive-tract/cervix/

Ticconi, C., Belmonte, A., Piccoine, E., & Rao, C. V. (2006). Feto-placental communication system with the myometrium in pregnancy and parturition: The role of hormones, neurohormones, inflammatory mediators, and locally active factors. *The Journal of Maternal-Fetal & Neonatal Medicine*, *19*(3), 125–133. doi:10.1080/14767050600555808 PMID:16690504

Verberg, M. F., Gillot, D. J., Al-Fardan, N., & Grudzinskas, J. G. (2005). Hyperemesis Gravidarum: A Literature Review. *Human Reproduction Update*, *11*(5), 527–539. doi:10.1093/humupd/dmi021 PMID:16006438

Walters, W. A., & Lim, Y. L. (1969). Cardiovascular dynamics in women receiving oral contraceptive therapy. *Lancet*, *2*(7626), 879–881. doi:10.1016/S0140-6736(69)92332-0 PMID:4186458

Weiss, E. R. (2020). *The role of the mucus plugs in pregnancy and labor*. Retrieved from https://www.verywellfamily.com/mucus-plug-and-role-in-labor-2759088

Whitlock, J. (2019). *The Function and Anatomy of the Uterus*. Retrieved from https://www.verywellhealth.com/uterus-location-function-female-anatomy-3157180

Wilson, R. D. (2017). *What bodily changes can you expect during pregnancy*. Retrieved from https://www.healthline.com/health/pregnancy/bodily-changes-during

Woodrow, J. P., Sharpe, C. J., Fudge, N. J., Hoff, A. O., Gagel, R. F., & Kovacs, C. S. (2006). Calcitonin plays a critical role in regulating skeletal mineral metabolism during lactation. *Endocrinology*, *147*(9), 4010–4021. doi:10.1210/en.2005-1616 PMID:16675524

World Bank. (1993). *World Development Report- Investing in Health*. Oxford University Press.

Yanamandra, N., & Chandraharan, E. (2012). Anatomical and physiological changes in pregnancy and their implications in clinical practice. In E. Chandraharan & S. Arulkumaran (Eds.), *Obstetric and Intrapartum Emergencies*. Published by Cambridge University Press. doi:10.1017/CBO9780511842153.002

Chapter 3
Essentials of Normal Pregnancy

ABSTRACT

Pregnancy is physiologically and nutritionally a highly demanding period. A pregnant woman prepares herself to meet the nutritional demands by increasing her own body fat deposits during pregnancy. The fetus inside the uterus of mother is like a parasite (i.e., it takes several nutrients that it requires from the mother, regardless of whether she has enough of them or not). However, it has been observed that women's diets among poor socio-economic groups during pre-pregnant, pregnant, and lactating periods are essentially similar. Consequently, widespread maternal malnutrition results in a high prevalence of infants with low birth weight and a very high maternal mortality rate. Extra diet is needed to improve the birth weight and increase deposits of fat in the maternal body. Adequate intake of nutritious diet is reflected in optimal weight gain of 10 to 12 kg during pregnancy. Some micronutrients are especially required in extra amounts to meet the physiological needs of this period. Hence, good nutrition must be ensured for optimum growth and development of children, adolescents, and women.

KEY FACTS

- One third of women of reproductive age in India are undernourished, with a Body Mass Index (BMI) of less than 18.5 Kg/m^2 (UNICEF, N.A.).

DOI: 10.4018/978-1-7998-4357-3.ch003

- There are various hormonal changes associated with menstruation, childbearing and menopause indicate that women are at an increased risk of anaemia and osteoporosis, thus requiring an increased intake of nutrients such as iron, calcium, magnesium, vitamin D, folate and other vitamins.
- The first 1000 days of a child's life, from conception to two years of age, is a critical window period of opportunities to address child stunting.
- It is essential that adequate nutrition reach women, regardless of whether they are pregnant or not, especially when the world strives towards reaching global targets of Sustainable Development Goals (SDG's) (United Nations, 2015).

INTRODUCTION

Pregnancy is, thus, a nutritionally demanding physiological state. Great importance lies in healthy nutrition during pregnancy and the following course of initial 1,000 days in light of the impact it has on the growth and the development of the baby, on the adequate development of the baby's brain, the immune system and the functional skills in its body. Healthy nutrition is the base for a healthy and balanced life, preventing ailments and promoting quality of life during the course of life. Recent research proves that the woman's' nutritional condition during pregnancy, the rate of her gaining weight and her nutritional habits can have an impact on the new-born's cognitive development, its tendency in becoming fatter during later life, heart and vascular diseases (Ministry of Health Israel, 2020).

Good nutrition, with a balance of macronutrients and micronutrients, at every stage of life is the key to human development. Good nutrition is vital to good health, disease prevention and essential for the optimum growth and development of children, adolescents and adults.

It is a common observation that women's diets from the poorer groups during pre-pregnant, pregnant and lactating periods are essentially similar. Consequently, there is widespread maternal malnutrition, results in a high prevalence of infants with low birth weight and a very high rate of maternal mortality. Thus, additional foods are needed to improve the birth weights and increase the body deposits of the mothers.

Article 47 of the Constitution of India is one of the directive principles which directs the state to raise the level of nutrition of the population. It also directs, as among its primary duties, to raise their standard of living and to improve the public health. In particular, the state shall endeavor to prohibit the use of intoxicating drinks and drugs that are injurious to health (Central Health Education Bureau, 2019).

The problem of under-nutrition runs in generations and is dependent on multifarious factors which include proper infant and young child feeding practices, completion of immunization schedule, institutional delivery as far as possible, regular check-ups for early detection of childhood development delays and subsequent follow up, consumption pattern in families affecting the life of adults and elderly. Food fortification (salt iodization, enrichment of flours etc.), regular administration of deworming drugs, iron supplement must be given to target the problem of anaemia. An access to safe drinking water and proper sanitation has an overriding effect on the overall status on the nutritional attainment in commensurate with the age and the physiological states such as pregnancy and lactation (Central Health Education Bureau, 2019).

Eating a well-balanced diet is important to stay healthy, maintain weight and remain energized but becomes more important in women because of hormonal changes associated with menstruation, child bearing and menopause which requires a higher intake of nutrients. Further, gender inequality, socio-cultural practices, lack of education, economic dependence and poor access to amenities make the situation even worse.

Nutrition

Nutrition is critical for the fulfillment of human rights for all populations but more especially for the most vulnerable population i.e. children, adolescent girls and women who are locked in a cycle of multiple deprivations between generations. It forms the basis of human development by declining their susceptibility to infection. This will ensure that associated morbidity, disability and mortality are reduced, cumulative lifelong learning capacities are enhanced and adult productivity is raised. It is essential to prevent under-nutrition as early as possible, throughout the life cycle, in order to prevent irreversible cumulative growth and development deficits which may compromise the health of mother and the child and their survival, achieve optimal learning outcomes in education and gender equality (Central Health Education Bureau (2019).

Malnutrition is one of the most persistent barriers to women's and girl's empowerment and socio-economic productivity and limits their capacity to grow, learn, earn and lead. It is essential that adequate nutrition reach them, regardless of whether they are pregnant or not, especially when the world strives towards reaching global targets of Sustainable Development Goals (SDG's) (United Nations, 2015).

Adolescents and Nutrition

Adolescents grow and develop physically, mentally and sexually at a very rapid pace. It is virtually impossible to overstate the role that good nutrition plays in the life of adolescent girls. She is increasing in height, bone and muscle mass whilst maturing almost every system and organ in her body. Good nutrition can optimize her physical and mental growth, give her the strength and focus for study, work, ward off disease and care for family (Central Health Education Bureau, 2019).

Well-nourished adolescent girls stay in the schools longer, achieve better learning outcomes, delay their marriage and first pregnancy, multiply their life options and advance their families as well as the development of the nation. Adolescence is the period to provide her an opportunity to overcome her nutritional deficiencies which may have occurred during childhood and to catch-up on growth due to deficit caused by the nutritional deprivation and also to establish good dietary behaviours. Adolescents should make healthy food and beverage choices; promote physical activity for the prevention of Iron Deficiency Anaemia (IDA) (Central Health Education Bureau, 2019).

A young adolescent girl is still a child; however, she will become a mother soon. Adolescent pregnancy is, therefore, associated with increased risk of maternal mortality and morbidity, stillbirths, neonatal deaths, premature births and babies born with low weight. Efforts are required to ensure that pregnant and lactating teenage mothers are adequately nourished.

Women and Nutrition

Similarly, in women, healthy foods help to reduce symptoms of pre-menstrual syndrome, boost fertility, makes pregnancy and nursing easier, eases the symptoms of menopause and keeps bones strong. As children, dietary needs of both boys and girls are largely similar but women begin to develop unique nutritional requirements when puberty begins. More physical and hormonal changes also occur with age, such that nutritional needs continue to develop making it critical to meet these changing needs of the growing bodies.

Women require fewer calories as compared to men but they have a much higher requirement for certain vitamins and minerals. Hormonal changes taking place during menstruation, childbearing, and menopause indicate that women are at an increased risk of anaemia, weakened bones, and osteoporosis, thereby requiring increased nutrient intakes such as iron, calcium, magnesium, vitamin D, folate as well as other vitamins and minerals. Often nutrient supplements are considered to be useful safeguard against nutrient deficiencies but they cannot compensate for an unbalanced or unhealthy diet (Smith et al, 2019).

There is an intergenerational malnutrition cycle by which a woman with iron deficiency anemia is likely to give birth to a baby with reduced birth weight. Babies with a low birth weight are likely to be wasted or stunted, and have a increased risk of morbidity and mortality and later in life, they are more prone to develop non-communicable diseases.

During pregnancy, anemia has a recognizable relation with the foetal outcome. There is an increased incidence of babies with low birth weight if the mother becomes anemic in her third trimester. There is again an increased incidence of preterm deliveries if in her second and third trimesters, the mother is anemic. Earlier supplementation with iron and maintaining optimal Hb (10–12 g / dl) throughout gestation has overall better outcome with regard to pre-term delivery and babies with low birth weight (Kumar et al, 2013).

In contrast, a mother becomes obese at the onset of her pregnancy, she is again at a higher risk of complications during pregnancy or delivery that could lead to pre-term delivery and thus a low birth weight for the newborn. Alternatively, there is more likelihood for her baby to have a higher birth weight at full term and an increased risk of child and adolescent obesity (Blanca et al, 2015).

One-third of reproductive-age women in India are undernourished, with a Body Mass Index (BMI) below 18.5 kg / m^2 (UNICEF, N.A.). It is a well-known fact that undernourished adolescent girls are more likely to become undernourished mothers, who are, in turn, more likely to give birth to babies with low birth weight. This cycle may be, further, compounded in young mothers, particularly adolescent girls, who begin early childbearing before they are fully grown and developed enough. Furthermore, mothers, who bear many children and give birth at short intervals between the pregnancies, are more susceptible to malnutrition. Child and maternal mortality and morbidity are examined in relation to the interval between pregnancies. Very little reliable information links child morbidity or maternal health detrimental to the spacing of short births. Child mortality evidence suggests very short intervals i.e. conceptions less than six months after a birth being detrimental to the survival of the second child and the mother (Winikoff, 1983).

From conception to two years of age, the first 1000 days of a child's life is a critical window of opportunity to address stunting among children. Mother's poor nutrition before and during pregnancy affects the foetus growth in the womb. Foetal stunting is mainly due to the mother's insufficient nutrition before conception and during the first trimester. Among Indian children, the main reason for stagnant levels of under-nutrition is poor nutrition of women both before and during pregnancy (Central Health Education Bureau, 2019).

Further, the first 1000 days of life from conception through pregnancy to child's second birthday present an important window of opportunity to improve child nutrition as well as good maternal nutrition and health are essential for optimal breastfeeding to the infant and child care. Exclusive breastfeeding, defined as the practice of giving only breast milk to the infant for the first six months of life without, in particular, any other food or water, has the single greatest preventive effect on child mortality. For timely and adequate complementary feeding, with particular attention to vitamin and mineral content, nutrient dense food is essential to lactating mothers (Central Health Education Bureau, 2019).

Thus, women and children's health and nutritional status are intimately linked. Improving women's and children's health, therefore, starts with ensuring women's health and nutritional status through her all stages of life. Further, female empowerment in respect of her health and nutritional status remains the key priority.

Requirement of Essential Nutrients

Nutrition is the science which interprets the interaction of nutrients and other substances present in food with respect to an organism's maintenance, growth, reproduction, health and disease. Nutrition includes ingestion, digestion, absorption, assimilation, biosynthesis, catabolism followed by excretion. Nutrients include protein, carbohydrate and fat as macronutrients and vitamins and minerals as micronutrients. The required amount of these nutrients varies with age, sex, activity and the physiological state of the body like pregnancy, lactation and any existing diseases (Central Health Education Bureau, 2019).

The gestation period is a time of rapid growth and evolution. Growth of the foetus and other developmental changes to facilitate its maintenance throughout pregnancy and delivery involve an increase in the nutritional demands of pregnant women.

Energy

During pregnancy, the mother needs more energy in the form of kilocalories, to supply the increased fuel demanded by the metabolic workload for both mother and the foetus and to spare protein for the added tissue building requirements. For these reasons, the pregnant mother must include more energy dense food in her diet.

For the proper management of an ideal body weight of women, it is essential that the total amount of calorie intake must not exceed the total calories consumed through metabolic processes during resting and the activity period. The additional energy is needed during pregnancy to support the growth of the fetus, placenta and maternal tissues as well as to meet the raised Basal Metabolic Rate (BMR). During the first and second trimesters, Basal metabolic rate increases by about 5 percent and by about 12 percent in the third trimester of pregnancy (Dakshayani and Murthy, 1964).

During pregnancy, the additional energy is required to support the growth of the foetus, placenta and the maternal tissues as well as to meet the increased Basal Metabolic Rate (BMR). Basal Metabolic Rate increases by about 5 percent during first and second trimester and by about 12 percent during the third trimester of pregnancy (Dakshayani and Murthy, 1964).

The total energy cost of pregnancy of a woman weighing 55 kg has been estimated to be 80,000 Kcal (WHO, 1973). Of this total energy requirement, about 36,000 Kcal is deposited as fat which is utilized subsequently during lactation. Based on these estimates, FAO/WHO Expert Group (WHO, 1965) recommended an extra daily allowance of 150 Kcal during first trimester and 350 Kcal during the rest of pregnancy. A direct estimate of energy estimate during normal pregnancy through indirect calorimetry has shown this to be around 27,000 Kcal (Emerson et al, 1972).

These levels of extra daily allowances of energy, however, would not allow for the deposition of fat, which is to be used during lactation to meet the additional energy needs for milk secretion. The earlier ICMR recommendations suggested an additional energy allowance of 300 Kcal/ day during pregnancy.

Experimental evidence both from India and outside India have demonstrated the beneficial effects of energy supplementation to pregnant women on birth weights of infants (Iyengar, 1967; Leihtiget al, 1975). On the basis of this evidence, the ICMR (1989) Committee felt that extra energy intake is desirable not only for the growth of foetus and the maternal tissues but also for the deposition of fat which can be utilized for meeting the increased energy demands during lactation. The committee, therefore, recommended an additional intake of 300 Kcal/ day during second and third trimester of pregnancy.

Active, large or nutritionally deficient women may require even more energy. The emphasis should always be on adequate energy to ensure the nutrient and energy needs of the rapidly growing foetus. Sufficient weight gain is vital to a successful pregnancy. However, an excess weight gain may pose risks and should be avoided. Increased complex carbohydrates and protein in the diet are the preferred sources of energy during pregnancy and lactation.

Protein

Protein is important for growth by the production, maintenance and repair of tissues in the body, besides the secretion of various enzymes, hormones and antibodies. However, when energy intake is insufficient, protein intake must be raised for meeting the energy requirements of the body. In an adult, dietary protein is essential to synthesize new proteins that will replace those which are constantly being broken down. For an adult, 1.0 per gram body weight of protein is adequate while adjusting for the lower quality of dietary proteins with 65 Net Protein Utilization (NPU), as per the RDA recommendations of ICMR (1978) (Gopalan and Narasinga, 1968).

Protein serves as the building blocks for the tremendous growth of body tissues during pregnancy. **Firstly**, it facilitates the rapid growth of foetus. During only 3 months, the increase in the size of the foetus from mere one cell to millions of cells in an infant of 3 kg indicate the requirement of relatively large amount of protein for such a rapid growth. **Secondly**, the mature placenta, the foetus lifeline to the mother, requires sufficient protein for its development as a vital and unique organ to sustain, support and nourish the foetus during growth. **Thirdly**, increased amount of protein is required for the growth of maternal tissues to support pregnancy and lactation. **Fourthly**, the mother's blood volume increases from 20 to 50 percent during pregnancy to nourish the foetus and support most of the increased metabolic workload which creates the need for more synthesis of blood components, especially hemoglobin and plasma protein. An increase in hemoglobin helps supply oxygen to the growing number of cells and plasma protein (albumin).

Plasma is the of watery, non-cellular blood component. During pregnancy, the plasma volume of the blood increases to help supply mother and baby with oxygen and nutrients. The total number of red blood cells may increase by 20 per cent but the amount of plasma increases even more, thereby resulting in dilution of red cells in the body. A pregnancy level of hemoglobin can naturally decrease to 10.5 gm / dL which is anemia in a normal pregnancy (Wedro, 2020).

Production increases to regulate blood volume though osmotic pressure. Adequate level of albumin also prevents an abnormal accumulation of water in tissues beyond the normal oedema of pregnancy. Moreover, amniotic fluid, which contains various proteins, surrounds the foetus during growth and guards it from shock and physical injury. Besides, an increased storage reserve of tissues is needed in the mother's body to prepare for the large amount of energy required during labour, delivery, immediate postpartum period and lactation (Nix, 2009).

During pregnancy, additional proteins are required for the synthesis of foetal tissue proteins. Protein requirements during pregnancy have been computed on the basis of nitrogen accretion for foetal growth and the expansion of maternal tissues. Based on an average body weight gain of 12 kg in a normal healthy well-nourished pregnant women, the daily nitrogen deposited during the three trimesters is estimated to be 0.1, 0.5, 0.9 gm respectively. After increasing by 50 percent to convert the factorial value into the physiological value for nitrogen accretion and 25 percent for individual variation, the safe level of intake in terms of a high quality protein during the three trimesters will be 1.2, 6.0 and 10.5 gm respectively. After adjusting for the dietary protein quality of Net Protein Utilization (NPU) of 65, the safe intake during pregnancy is 15 gm per day in addition to her normal protein requirement (ICMR, 1989).

The complete protein foods of high biological value include egg, milk, cheese, meat (beef, poultry, fish and pork) and soya products. Other incomplete proteins from plant sources such as legumes and grains contribute additional secondary amount of protein.

Fat

Fats are a concentrated and rich source of energy and increase the energy density of the diet. Fat in the diet also helps in the absorption of B-Carotene and other Vitamins soluble in fat. Dietary fat provides essential fatty acids

(EFA) that are the functional components of the membrane lipids and perform various other important metabolic functions.

The diets of even poor people which consists of predominantly of cereals and have little or no visible fat contains significant quantities of invisible fat. The invisible fat from cereals and pulses alone contribute as much as 6 en% or 16 grams of invisible fat in an adult diet that provides 2400 Kcal per day (Ghafoorunissa, 1989). In average Indian diets in many parts of the country, the total visible plus invisible fat contributes about 15 percent of the dietary energy, though in the diets of poor income groups, this reduces to about 10 percent of dietary energy. Continuous intake of daily diets providing an average of about 15 percent of energy from fat does not lead to any fat deficiency (Achaya, 1987). A daily Indian diet which provides 2400 Kcal will thus carry about 40 grams of fat per day, out of which 25gm will be invisible fat and 15 grams of visible fat.

It is recommended that fat intake totals should be no more than 30 percent of the total calorie intake. Polyunsaturated fat should be reduced to less than 10 percent of the calories and saturated and trans-fats together should be reduced to less than 10 percent of the fat intake. The remainder of the fat intake should be monounsaturated fat. These fats are present mainly in deep fried fast foods and processed foods made up of margarine.

- ***Trans-Fats:*** These fats are made artificially through a chemical process. This solidifies the oil and limits the ability of the body to control its cholesterol. These fats are treated as hazardous to health.
- ***Saturated Fats:*** Saturated fat is present in foods such as butter and beef fat. Such fats are rich in palmitic and stearic fatty acids.
- ***Monounsaturated Fats:*** This is found mainly in chicken fat and vegetable oils such as olive, canola and peanut oils. These fats are rich in oleic fatty acids.
- ***Polyunsaturated Fats:*** This group includes Omega-3 and Omega-6 essential fatty acids (EFA). These are found in high levels in fish oil, vegetable and nut oils. These fats contain linoleic and linolenic fatty acids.

The essential fatty acids (EFA) linoleic and linolenic fatty acids cannot be synthesized in the body and have to be supplied through dietary fat. Dietary fat with an equal proportion of saturated, monounsaturated and polyunsaturated fatty acids components have been considered as desirable.

Linoleic and linolenic fatty acids are the essential fatty acids (EFA) which are further metabolized in the body into other fatty acids of long chain length and unsaturation that perform important biological functions in the body. Some of these are a part of cell structures while others perform a specific role in vision and functions of the central nervous system.

Linoleic and linolenic fatty acids are also converted into prostaglandins, thromboxanes and prostacyclines that perform extremely crucial functions in areas such as blood pressure regulation, viscosity of the blood, muscle contraction, pain relief, male fertility and female contraception as well as the normal delivery.

The linoleic requirement during pregnancy is 4.5 en%. Taking into account the contribution from the invisible fat, 12.5 en % visible fats would meet the essential fatty acids (EFA) requirement. The corresponding visible fat intake will be 30 gm per day. This level of fat intake would also provide the necessary calorie density to the diet of pregnant women (ICMR, 1989).

Carbohydrates

Carbohydrates are the main instant source of energy for both the mother and the baby. A close association exists between the blood sugar (glucose) level of mother and that of baby's. Glucose is the main energy source for the baby. Carbohydrates should contribute to total calories to the extent of at least 55 percent. The brain is the specialized organ of the body that depends primarily on glucose for its energy. The brain requires about 100 grams of glucose as fuel for providing energy. Under certain conditions, the body compensates for the reduced intake of carbohydrates by using alternative pathways, such as burning of fatty acids. During pregnancy, complex carbohydrates should be preferred source of energy.

Vitamins and Minerals

During pregnancy, an increase in several vitamins and minerals is needed in order to meet the greater structural and metabolic requirements. Several of these essential substances have key roles in pregnancy and require special attention.

Iron

Iron is one of the keys to good health and energy levels prior to menopause. In India, iron deficiency anaemia is quite widespread, the prevalence varying from 45 percent in adult males to 70 percent or more in women and children (Working Group on Fortification of Salt with Iron, 1982). While the main etiological factor of the dietary iron deficiency, folate deficiency also contributes to anaemia among young children and pregnant women.

There is a two- to three-fold increase in the requirement for iron during pregnancy. This increase is meant not only for haemoglobin synthesis but also for the growing foetus and also for certain enzymes production. This is also accompanied by a 10- to 20-fold increase in folate requirements and a two-fold increase in the requirement for vitamin B_{12} (Soma-Pillay, 2016).

During pregnancy, iron requirements can be calculated from iron needs for the growth of the foetal, maternal tissues expansion, including red cell mass, iron content in placenta as well as blood loss during parturition. In addition to the basic requirement of iron, these additional requirements should be added. Yet, the menstrual loss is saved during pregnancy. The mean requirement is not raised during the first trimester. It is same as the usual requirement of 0.7 mgm while the daily requirement is 3.3 milligrams and 5.0 milligrams respectively during the second and third trimesters of pregnancy (ICMR, 1989).

Iron absorption from Indian diets based on cereals and millets is quite low. It ranges from 2-5 percent depending upon the type of staple, the absorption being highest from rice based diets and lowest from diets based on millets like ragi. Iron absorption from the daily diet determined by multiple tagging of different meals give an average value of 3 percent (2.6-3.6) which is 5 percent for pregnant women (Narasinga et al, 1983). This makes the dietary iron requirement on a mixed cereal diet to be 37.5 grams per day for pregnant women.

Consuming foods high in vitamin C along with dietary sources of iron enhances the body's ability to absorb and use the low bioavailable iron. In addition, avoiding foods that inhibit iron absorption such as whole grain cereals, legumes, tea and coffee, with meals that provide sufficient iron is recommended. Since the increased requirement of pregnancy is difficult to meet with the iron content of a typical mixed diet, daily iron supplements are often recommended (Kaiser and Allen, 2002).

Iron rich foods include red meat, chicken, turkey, pork, fish, spinach, beans, lentils and some ready-to-eat cereals. Iron obtained from plant-based sources is more readily absorbed by body when taken along with foods rich in vitamin C.

Folic Acid

Folate builds mature RBC's throughout pregnancy and is particularly needed during the peri-conception period i.e. from 2 months before conception to 6 weeks of gestation so as to ensure healthy embryonic tissue development and prevent the malformation of the neural tube (McLone, 2003). This tissue forms during the critical period from 17 to 30 days of gestation and grows into the mature infant's spinal column and its network of nerves.

The primary function of folic acid is related to the synthesis of a number of metabolites in the body being transferred from single carbonin. In addition to vitamin B12, folic acid is linked with nucleic acid synthesis. Folic acid undergoes a series of metabolic conversions to its diverse co-enzymic forms after its absorption. Folic acid deficiency, if prolonged and severe, leads to abnormal haemopoiesis, leading to megaloblastic anaemia which readily responds to the administration of this vitamin (Nix, 2009).

When women reach child bearing age, they need to have enough folate (folic acid) to help decrease the effect of birth defects. The requirement of folic acid during pregnancy is known to increase and the additional amounts needed have been estimated to range between 150-300 micrograms per day (WHO, 1985).

Findings of studies carried out on Indian women have recommended that requirement of folate is between 200 and 300 micrograms during pregnancy so as to maintain plasma and red cell folate levels within the normal range (Iyengar, 1971). Birth weights were found to be more for infants born to mothers receiving 300 micrograms of folate per day during pregnancy as compared to those born to mothers receiving 100 or 200 micrograms per day. These findings recommend that pregnant women need 300 microgram of additional folic acid daily. It is difficult to provide this amount through food and the additional needs may have to be met through supplements of medicinal folate.

For those women, who are not pregnant, require is 400 micrograms of folate per day. Adequate amounts of foods that naturally contain folate like citrus fruits, leafy greens, beans and peas should be included in the daily diet that will facilitate an increased intake of this B vitamin. This is especially true for women who are pregnant or breastfeeding, since their daily need for folate is higher i.e. 600 and 500 micrograms per day respectively (Food and Nutrition Board, 1999).

All enriched flours and grain products, as well as fortified cereals have well absorbed form of dietary folic acid. Other natural sources include liver, dark green leafy vegetables, legumes (black beans and kidney beans), soyabean, wheat germ, orange juice, asparagus and broccoli.

Calcium and Vitamin D

It is essential to have a good supply of calcium, along with phosphorus, magnesium and vitamin D, for the development of bones and teeth of the foetus as well as meet the mother's body needs. Calcium is also required for proper clotting of blood. During pregnancy, the physiologic changes occur in the mother's absorption capacity to help meet the needs of some nutrients e.g. calcium and zinc are both are significantly more bioavailable during pregnancy (Vargas Zapata et al, 2004; Donangelo et al, 2005). The body's enhanced capability to absorb and retain these nutrients from the diet during pregnancy helps the mother meet her nutrient needs and those of the growing foetus.

For healthy bones and teeth, women need to each a variety of calcium rich foods every day and to reduce the risk of osteoporosis, a bone disease in which the bones become weak and break easily. Though small in quantity, non-skeletal calcium has an important role to play in neuromuscular excitation, clotting of the blood, permeability of the membrane, etc. Calcium's importance for these functions is reflected in the precision of regulation of plasma calcium. In bones, calcium plays an important role in maintaining this level, even in the face of inadequate dietary calcium.

Adults require calcium to replace the calcium lost from the body through urine, stool, bile and the sweat. In adults, this loss is estimated to be 700 milligrams per day. The body can, however, reduce this loss on low calcium intake through an adaptation process involving reduced excretion (Shenolikar and Narasinga, 1968). About 20-30 percent of the calcium in the diet is absorbed and such absorption is greatly facilitated by the intake of vitamin D. however, additional calcium is required during pregnancy for foetal growth and skeletal development.

To maintain its physiological processes, the average foetus requires about 30 grams of calcium. During the third trimester, most of this calcium is transferred to the foetus which is mainly derived from an increased dietary absorption of calcium by the mother (Kovacs, 2006). During pregnancy, the total serum calcium concentration falls. This is caused by a decrease in serum albumin levels due to haemodilution, which leads to a decline in the albumin-bound calcium fraction. However, the important physiological fraction, serum ionized calcium, remains unchanged (Woodrow et al, 2006).

Therefore, during pregnancy, maternal serum calcium levels are maintained. The needs of the foetus are met through increased intestinal absorption, which increase two-fold after 12 weeks of gestation. Yet, the peak calcium demand is only during third trimester. This early increase in absorption of calcium may enable the skeleton of mother to store calcium beforehand (Davison et al, 1989).

There is an increase in the serum levels of 25-hydroxyvitamin D. This is metabolized further into 1.25-dihydroxyvitamin D. The rise in 1.25-dihydroxyvitamin D level is directly responsible for the rise in intestinal calcium absorption (Woodrow et al, 2006).

Increased absorption of calcium is closely associated with an increase in urine calcium excretion and such changes commence at 12 weeks of gestation. The urinary calcium values are low or normal during fasting periods, thus confirming that hyper-calciuria is the outcome of increased calcium absorption (Kovacs, 2006). Therefore pregnancy is a risk factor for kidney stones.

Various foods rich in calcium include low-fat or fat-free milk, yogurt and cheese, sardines, tofu, foods fortified with calcium, including juices and cereals. It is also important to have adequate amount of vitamin D in the diet. The need for both calcium and vitamin D rises with the ageing of women. Good vitamin D sources include fatty fish such as salmon, eggs, and fortified foods and beverages, such as some yogurts and juices. The best source of vitamin D is sunlight. The mother's exposure to sunlight increases endogenous synthesis of vitamin D as well. Lactose intolerant women or vegetarians can obtain adequate vitamin D from fortified soya or rice milk products.

Nutrient Supplementation (Central Health Education Bureau, 2019)

- ***National Iron Plus Initiative:*** To provide for the supplementation of iron and folic acid for pregnant and lactating women and children in the age group of 6 to 60 months as well as adolescents both in and out of school as well as women in reproductive age groups, National Iron Plus Initiative has been launched by Government of India.
- ***National Iodine Deficiency Disorder Control Programme:*** In order to combat the problem of Iodine Deficiency Disorder (IDD) in India, National Iodine Deficiency Disorder Control programme (NIDDCP) was launched. It has been made mandatory to supply iodized salt instead of common salt under this program.

- ***Dietary Supplementation:*** Integrated Child Development Services (ICDS) scheme was launched in 1975 with the objective to improve the nutritional and health status of children, pregnant and nursing mothers. Supplementary nutrition is provided to children below the age of six years, adolescents, pregnant and nursing mothers.
- ***Poshan Abhiyan:*** Poshan Abhiyan, an overreaching scheme for all around attack towards proper nourishment, envisages targeting stunting, under-nutrition, low birth weight in children, anaemia in children, adolescents and pregnant and lactating women to combat malnutrition with a 360 degree approach. The program also envisages targeting the growing issue of over-nutrition in children, adolescents and adults by promotion of nutritionally balanced diets.

There are significant health benefits for peri-menopausal and menopausal women in maintaining optimum levels of vitamins and nutrients such as vitamin K2, vitamin D, calcium, omega-3, vitamins B, zinc, magnesium, and iron. Supplementation with phyto-estrogens could also have a significant role to play in balancing the decline in endogenous estrogen (Ward, 2017).

To promote the notion of healthy nutrition for the population, a holistic approach is required. In order to make people aware of the importance of healthy nutrition, it is necessary to keep in mind the cultural diversity in food habits and the earning capacity of the population, multi-sectoral innovative approaches should be adopted to involve all age groups. In various schools, family and childcare centres, the initiative should be taken right from childhood so that the foundation of healthy eating habits is laid at the right age and can also be further propagated in future generations. Policy making should ensure the availability of nutritious food at low cost, as well as mobilizing community and health education.

Immunization

Maternal immunization offers considerable health benefits to both pregnant women and the foetus. Vaccine-preventable diseases lead to significant morbidity and mortality among infants of the maternal, neonatal and young children. There are some infections of severe nature that they not only damage the pregnancy but also harm the foetus during pregnancy or the newborn after delivery. Vaccination can protect such complications. For pregnant mothers, vaccinations are, therefore, very important. Vaccines strengthen body's immune systems that can combat serious infectious diseases (Verma et al, 2016).

A vaccine provides protection to the mother's body from infections and during pregnancy, this immunity is transferred to the foetus. This immunity protects the newborn from infections for the first few months of life until the baby gets his or her own immunization. Vaccination also safeguard mothers from a severe illness that might adversely affect her future pregnancies. However, fetus receiving any risk after mother's vaccination during pregnancy is theoretical (Verma et al, 2016).

Tetanus Toxoid Vaccine

Severe maternal morbidity and neonatal mortality can be caused by tetanus. It is a life-threatening bacterial disease caused by toxin of bacterium, named *Clostridium Tetani*, which is frequently present in the soil. Bacteria of tetanus enter the body by open wound. It may well be a small prick or scratch on the skin, although tetanus infection is more frequent when a deep puncture wound such as bite, cut, burn or ulcer occurs (Park, 2014).

The nervous system of a person is affected by tetanus, and if untreated, it can be fatal. In newborns, infection of the unhealed umbilical stump causes neonatal tetanus, especially when the stump is cut with a non-sterile instrument. Vaccination can only prevent tetanus (Silveira et al, 1995; Verma and Khanna, 2012).

The vaccine of tetanus contains toxoids which are non-infectious. During pregnancy, tetanus toxoids are quite safe and are given to prevent neonatal tetanus in many countries of the world. The World Health Organization (WHO) has reported that more than 200,000 newborns every year are killed by neonatal tetanus; nearly all these deaths occur in developing countries, while in developed nations, these are very rare (World Health organization, 2015).

The National Immunization Schedule in India recommends the 2 doses of tetanus toxoid (TT) for unknown immunization status of pregnant women, i.e. the first dose of tetanus toxoid should be given as soon as pregnancy is detected, the second dose of tetanus toxoid should be given after 4 to 6 weeks so as to maximize the maternal antibody response and passive antibody transfer to the infant. If a mother has received 2 dozes of TT during her last pregnancy and she becomes pregnant again within 3 years, then only one TT dose is recommended and this dose acts as booster dose. Some experts recommend administering the second dose of the vaccine 4 weeks before the expected delivery date. WHO also recommends that a third dose of vaccine should be given 6 months after the second one to provide at least 5 years of protection. The antibodies formed in mother's body are transferred to the foetus after TT vaccination which protect the newborn for a few months after birth. Vaccination of TT also prevents premature delivery or birth (Verma, 2014). The American Congress of Obstetricians and Gynecologists recommends the use of tetanus immune globulin as there is no evidence of tetanus immunoglobin adversely affecting the foetus (American College of Obstetricians and Gynecologists (ACOG), 1993).

Influenza Vaccine

Influenza may result in serious illness in pregnant women as compared to women who are not pregnant. There is a change in the immune system, heart and lungs during pregnancy which renders pregnant women more vulnerable to severe illness requiring hospitalizations and even influenza causing death. During pregnancy, influenza infection also gives the unborn babies a greater chance of serious problems, including premature labor and delivery. Women who are at increased risk for influenza hospitalization are those in the second and third trimesters of pregnancy. This is why, routine inactivated influenza vaccine is recommended for all women who are pregnant during the influenza season (in any trimester) (Centers for Disease Control and Prevention (CDC), 2013).

For the control of seasonal influenza, the available inactivated influenza vaccines are safe and efficacious. Such vaccines can prevent significant morbidity and mortality among pregnant women (World Health organization, 2003).

Live attenuated influenza vaccine in the form of an intranasal spray is available but this is not recommended for pregnant women. Maternal influenza immunization offers demonstrable benefits for women and their newborns from disease prevention and is a critically important component in pregnancy. Pregnant women should be advised on the advantages of the influenza vaccine for themselves and their foetus (Verma et al, 2012).

Hepatitis B Vaccine

Infection with hepatitis B is a serious infection which causes liver inflammation. Infection with hepatitis B in a pregnant woman may result in severe morbidity for the mother and may increase the likelihood of premature birth. However, there is no evidence indicating that infection with hepatitis B is not associated with increased rates of abortion, stillbirth or congenital fetal malformation (Verma et al, 2011).

Thus, the biggest challenge is the vertical transmission i.e. transmission of infection from mother to foetus. As many as 70 to 90 percent of babies remain chronically infected with hepatitis B into their adult lives, they develop liver cirrhosis and hepatocellular carcinoma later on (Singh, 2004).

In view of the such high risks of infection with hepatitis B and the safety and efficacy (sero-conversion 90 to 100 percent) of the Hepatitis B vaccine in the prevention of infection with hepatitis B, it is recommended that high-risk pregnant women receive the Hepatitis B vaccine. The vaccine for hepatitis B is an inactivated (recombinant) virus vaccine. Since it is composed of non-infectious surface antigen particles of hepatitis B, it should not cause an increased risk to pregnant women (Margolis, 2005).

Globally, many studies have confirmed that there are no adverse pregnancy outcomes reported after vaccinated with HepB vaccine during pregnancy (Reddy et al, 1994; Grosheide, et al, 2012). Pregnancy is, thus, not a contraindication to vaccination. However, pregnant women who are at high risk for acquiring Hepatitis B infection, the Hepatitis B vaccine should be administered to them during pregnancy (Margolis, 2005; Canadian Immunization Guide, 2006).

A mother with HBsAg-positive should be carefully monitored to ensure that the infant receives hepatitis B immunoglobulin and starts the vaccine schedule for hepatitis B no later than 12 hours after birth. It must be ensured that the infant completes the recommended vaccine schedule of hepatitis B. The passive immunization of pregnant women with immune globulin preparations does not present a known risk for the foetus.

Hepatitis A Vaccine

Globally, an estimated 1.4 million cases of hepatitis A virus (HAV) infection occurs every year World Health organization (2014). It has been reported by Integrated Disease Surveillance Program of the National Center for Disease Control that 290,000 cases of acute viral hepatitis were identified in the year 2013. Its mode of infection is through fecal-oral route by the intake of contaminated food or water (National Centre for Disease Control, 2014).

Hepatitis A vaccines are derived from viruses grown in diploid cell cultures and are formalin inactivated (Gall, 1999; Verma and Khanna, 2012). During pregnancy, however, safety of hepatitis A vaccination has not been determined. The risk to the developing fetus is expected to be low because hepatitis A vaccine is produced from inactivated virus. Therefore, theoretical risks of vaccination to pregnant women, who may be at risk of exposure, should be weighed against the risk of hepatitis A infection. Finally, if a pregnant woman is exposed to infection with hepatitis A, it is strongly recommended to give her immune globulin. The immunoglobulin is considered safe and is more than 85 percent effective in preventing acute infection from hepatitis during pregnancy (Atkinson, 2002; Centre for Disease Control, 1999).

Live attenuated virus is a vaccine that can pass through the placenta and cause the foetus to become infected by viruses. This is the reason that most live attenuated vaccines such as measles, mumps, rubella, varicella, meningococcal, human papilloma virus (HPV) and pneumococcal polysaccharide vaccine, oral polio vaccine (OPV), inactivated polio vaccine (IPV), typhoid vaccine, cholera vaccine, plague vaccine, Japanese encephalitis vaccine are strongly contraindicated among pregnant women.

In India, vaccination during pregnancy is a cost-effective strategy for improving the outcomes of pregnancy. Inactivated virus, bacterial or toxoid vaccination during pregnancy is theoretical risk to a developing foetus. However, the live vaccine definitely represents a theoretical risk to a developing foetus.Thus, all live vaccines during pregnancy should be avoided.

During pregnancy, common vaccination barriers include lack of awareness regarding its advantages and lack of vaccine safety concerns. The government should include those vaccines in the routine immunization schedule in the developing country like India where people cannot afford these vaccines.

Physical Activity

Moderate physical activity on regular basis has shown proven results in terms of marked benefits for both the mother and the foetus. The benefits of moderate physical activity to mothers include improved cardio-vascular function, limited pregnancy weight gain, decreased musculo-skeletal discomfort, lower oedema, reduced rate of gestational diabetes and hypertension and less complicated labour. Benefits to the growing foetus include decreased fat mass, improved tolerance to stress and an advanced neuro-behavioural maturation.

American College of Obstetricians and Gynecologists (2002) (ACOG) has recommended that pregnant women who are free of medical or obstetric complications should follow the American College of Sports Medicine – Centers for Disease Control and Prevention general guidelines for physical activity. Such women should engage in more than or equal to 30 minutes of moderate physical activity per day, if possible (American College of Sports Medicine, 2006).

For active women with normal pregnancies, nearly 30 minutes of moderate physical activity per day is recommended which is accompanied by improved cardiovascular fitness, with no adverse effects on foetal condition or labour and the delivery outcomes. Furthermore, this recommended level of physical activity can contribute to a reduction in both the duration of the second stage of labour and the incidence of operational delivery (Melzer et al, 2010).

CONCLUSION

Pregnancy involves a fundamental interaction of the three distinct yet unified biological entities; the foetus, placenta and the mother. The increasing nutritional needs of the foetus and the placenta are also reflected through the maternal needs. Moreover, the optimum gain in weight varies with the normal nutritional status as well as the weight of the women, with an objective of 10 to 12 kg weight gain for a woman of average weight. Sufficient weight gain is important during pregnancy to support the rapid growth of foetus taking place. However, the nutritional quality of diet of the pregnant mother is as significant as the actual weight gain. Unusual or irregular eating habits, age, parity, pre-pregnancy weight status are among the many related conditions that put pregnant women at risk of complications.

REFERENCES

Achaya, K. T. (1987). Fat status of Indians: A Review. *Journal of Scientific and Industrial Research (New Delhi, India)*, *46*, 112.

American College of Obstetricians and Gynecologists. (2002). Exercise during pregnancy and the postpartum period: ACOG committee opinion no. 267. *Obstetrics and Gynecology*, *99*, 171–173. PMID:11777528

American College of Obstetricians and Gynecologists (ACOG). (1993). Immunization during pregnancy. Technical bulletin number 160- October 1991. *International Journal of Gynaecology and Obstetrics*, *40*(1), 69-79. doi:10.1016/0020-7292(93)90778-U

American College of Sports Medicine. (2006). *ACSM's guidelines for exercise testing and prescription* (*7th ed.*). Lippincott Williams & Wilkins.

Atkinson, W. (2002). Epidemiology and prevention of vaccine-preventable diseases. *Centers for Disease Control and Prevention.*

Branca, F., Piwoz, E., Schultink, W., & Sullivan, M. L. (2015). Nutrition and health in women, children and adolescents girls. *British Medical Journal, 351*. Advance online publication. doi:10.1136/bmj.h4173 PMID:26371218

Canadian Immunization Guide. (2006). (7th ed.). Ottawa: Public Health Agency of Canada; Health Agency of Canada. Available from: www.phac-aspc.gc.ca/publicat/cig-gci/index-eng.php\

Central Health Education Bureau. (2019). *Healthy India Initiative*. New Delhi: Directorate General of Health Services, Ministry of Health and Family Welfare, Government of India.

Centers for Disease Control and Prevention (CDC). (2013). Prevention and control of seasonal influenza with vaccines. Recommendations of the Advisory Committee on Immunization Practices —United States, 2013–2014..

Centre for Disease Control. (1999). Prevention of hepatitis A through active or passive immunization: Recommendations of the Advisory Committee on Immunization Practices (ACIP). Morbidity and Mortality Weekly Reports (MMWR). *Recommendations and Reports*, *48*(RR-12), 1–37.

Dakshayani, R., & Ramana Murthy, P. S. V. (1964). Basal metabolism and creatinine excretion in different physiological groups. *The Indian Journal of Medical Research*, *52*, 1159. PMID:14247617

Davison, J. M., Sheills, E. A., Barron, W. M., Robinson, A. G., & Lindheimer, M. D. (1989). Changes in the metabolic clearance of vasopressin and in plasma vasopressinase throughout human pregnancy. *The Journal of Clinical Investigation*, *83*(4), 1313–1318. doi:10.1172/JCI114017 PMID:2703533

Donangelo, C. M., Vargas Zapata, C. L., Woodhouse, L. R., Shames, D. M., Mukherjea, R., & King, J. C. (2005). Zinc absorption and kinetics during pregnancy and lactation in Brazilian women. *The American Journal of Clinical Nutrition*, *82*(1), 118–124. doi:10.1093/ajcn/82.1.118 PMID:16002809

Emerson, K., Saxena, B. N., & Poindexter, E. L. (1972). Caloric cost of normal Pregnancy. *Obstetrics and Gynecology*, *40*, 786. PMID:4636907

Food and Nutrition Board, Institute of Medicine. (1999). *Dietary reference intakes for thiamin, riboflavin,niacin, vitamin B_6, folate, vitamin B_{12}, pantothenic acid, biotin and choline*. National Academic Press.

Gall, S. A. (1999). Immunizations in the adult female patient. *The Female Patient, 24*, 53–59.

Ghafoorunissa. (1989). Fat and fatty acid content of cereals and pulsesand their relevance to Indian Diets. *European Journal of Clinical Nutrition, 43*, 275.

Gopalan, C., & Narasinga Rao, B. S. (1968). *Dietary Allowances for Indians*. Special Report Series No. 60, Indian Council of medical research, Hyderabad.

Grosheide, P.M., & Schalm, S.W., Van Os, H.C., Fetter, W.P. & Heijtink, R.A. (2012). Immune response to hepatitis B vaccine in pregnant women receiving post-exposure prophylaxis. *European Journal of Obstetrics, Gynecology, and Reproductive Biology, 8*(5), 1–4. PMID:8365536

Indian Council of Medical Research. (1989). *Nutritive Value of Indian Foods*. National Institute of Nutrition.

Iyengar, L. (1971). Folic Acid Requirement of Indian Pregnant Women. *American Journal of Obstretics and Gynecology, 111*, 13.

Iyengar, L. (1967). Effect of dietary supplements late in pregnancy on the expectant mother and her newborn. *Indian Journal of Medical Research, 55*, 85.

Kaiser, L. L., & Allen, L. (2002). Position of the American Dietetic Association: Nutrition and lifestyle for a healthy pregnancy outcome. *Journal of the American Dietetic Association, 102*(10), 1479–1490. doi:10.1016/S0002-8223(02)90327-5 PMID:12396171

Kovacs, C. S. (2006). Calcium metabolism during pregnancy and lactation. *NCBI Bookshelf*. https://www.ncbi.nlm.nih.gov/books/NBK279173/

Kumar, K. J., Asha, N., Murthy, D. S., Sujatha, M., & Manjunath, V. (2013). Maternal anemia in various trimesters and its effect on newborn weight and maturity: An observational study. *International Journal of Preventive Medicine, 4*(2), 193–199. PMID:23543625

Leihtig, A., & Habicht, J.P., Delgado, H., Klien, R.E., Yarbrough, C., & Mortorell, R. (1975). Effect of food supplementation during pregnancy on birth weight. *Pediatrics, 56*, 508. PMID:1165955

Margolis, H. S., Fiore, A. E., Brink, E. W., Goldstein, S. T., & Wang, S. A. (2005). A comprehensive immunization strategy to eliminate transmission of hepatitis B virus infection in the United States: Recommendations of the Advisory Committee on Immunization Practices (ACIP) part 1: immunization of infants, children, and adolescents. *MMWR Recomm Rep.B*, *54*(RR-16), 1–23. PMID:16371945

McLone, D. G. (2003). The etiology of neural tube defects: The role of folic acid. *Child's Nervous System*, *19*(7-8), 537–539. doi:10.100700381-003-0793-2 PMID:12920544

Melzer, K., Schutz, Y., Soehnchen, N., Othenin-Girard, V., Martinez de Tejada, B., Irion, O., Boulvain, M., & Kayser, B. (2010). Effects of recommended levels of physical activity on pregnancy outcomes. *American Journal of Obstetrics and Gynecology*, *202*(3), 266.e1–266.e6. doi:10.1016/j.ajog.2009.10.876 PMID:20022583

Ministry of Health, State of Israel. (2020). *Proper nutrition during pregnancy*. Retrieved fromhttps://www.health.gov.il/English/Topics/Pregnancy/during/Pages/proper_nutrition_during_pregnancy.aspx

Narasinga Rao, B. S., Vijayasarathy, C., & Prabhavati, T. (1983). Iron Absorption from habitual Diets of Indians studied by Extrinsic Tag Technique. *The Indian Journal of Medical Research*, *77*, 648. PMID:6618538

National Centre for Disease Control. (2014). *Newsletter quarterly newsletter from the National Centre for Disease Control*, *3*(1), 1-3.

Nix, S. (2009). *William's Basic Nutrition Diet Therapy*. Elesevier Inc.

Park, K. (2014). Epidemiology of communicable diseases. In Park's Textbook of Preventive and Social medicine. Jabalpur, India: Banarsidas Bhanot Publishers.

Reddy, P. A., Gupta, I., & Ganguly, N. K. (1994). Hepatitis-B vaccination in pregnancy: Safety and immunogenic response in mothers and antibody transfer to neonates. *Asia-Oceania Journal of Obstetrics and Gynaecology*, *20*(4), 361–365. doi:10.1111/j.1447-0756.1994.tb00482.x PMID:7832667

Shenolikar, I. S., & Narasinga Rao, B. S. (1968). Influence of Dietary Protein on Calcium Metabolismin young rats. *The Indian Journal of Medical Research*, *56*, 1412. PMID:5703360

Silveira, C. M., Caceres, V. M., Dutra, M. G., Lopes-Camelo, J., & Castilla, E. E. (1995). Safety of tetanus toxoid in pregnant women: A hospital-based casecontrol study of congenital anomalies. *Bulletin of the World Health Organization*, *73*(5), 605–608. PMID:8846486

Singh, S. P. (2004). Hepatitis B immunization: FAQs. *Hepatitis B Annual*, *1*(1), 240–248.

Smith, M., Segal, J., & Robinson, L. (2019). *Diet and Nutrition Tips for Women*. Retrieved from https://www.helpguide.org/articles/healthy-eating/diet-and-nutrition-tips-for-women.htm

Soma-Pillay, P., Nelson-Piercy, C., Tolppanen, H., Mebazaa, A., & Mebazaa, A. (2016). Physiological Changes in Pregnancy. *Cardiovascular Journal of Africa*, *27*(2), 89-94. https://www.ncbi.nlm.nih.gov/pmc/articles/PMC4928162/

UNICEF. (n.d.). *Child Survival Growth and Development: Women Nutrition*. UNICEF.

United Nation. (2015). *Sustainable Development Goals*. Retrieved from https://www.un.org/development/desa/disabilities/envision2030.html

Vargas Zapata, C. L., Donangelo, C. M., Woodhouse, L. R., Abrams, S. A., Spencer, E. M., & King, J. C. (2004). Calcium homeostasis during pregnancy and lactation in Brazilian women with low calcium intakes: A longitudinal study. *The American Journal of Clinical Nutrition*, *80*(2), 417–422. doi:10.1093/ajcn/80.2.417 PMID:15277164

Verma, R. (2014). Immunization. In Manual of Practical Community Medicine. Chandigarh, India: Saurabh Medical Publisher.

Verma, R. & Khanna, P. (2012). Tetanus toxoid vaccine: Elimination of neonatal tetanus in selected states of India. *Human Vaccines Immunotherapeutics*, *8*(10), 1-4. doi:10.1016/0028-2243(93)90164-8

Verma, R., & Khanna, P. (2012). Hepatitis A vaccine should receive priority in National Immunization Schedule in India. *Human Vaccines & Immunotherapeutics*, *8*(9), 1–3. doi:10.4161/hv.20475 PMID:22854671

Verma, R., Khanna, P., & Chawla, S. (2012). Influenza Vaccine: An effective preventive vaccine for developing countries. *Human Vaccines & Immunotherapeutics*, *8*(5), 1–4. doi:10.4161/hv.19516 PMID:22634439

Verma, R., Khanna, P., & Suraj Chawla, S. P. (2011). Hepatitis B vaccine in the national immunization schedule: A preventive step in India. *Human Vaccines & Immunotherapeutics*, *7*(12), 1–2. PMID:22134433

Ward, G. (2017). *Women's Health Focus – Nutrition during Peri-Menopause and Menopause*. Retrieved from https://www.nutri-facts.org/en_US/news/womens-health-focus-nutrition-during-peri-menopause-and-menopause.html

Wedro, B. (2020). *Anemia during Pregnancy*. Retrieved from https://www.medicinenet.com/anemia_in_pregnancy/views.htm

Winikoff, B. (1983). The Effects of Birth Spacing on Child and Maternal Health. *Studies in Family Planning*, *14*(10), 231–245. doi:10.2307/1965748 PMID:6648993

Woodrow, J. P., Sharpe, C. J., Fudge, N. J., Hoff, A. O., Gagel, R. F., & Kovacs, C. S. (2006). Calcitonin plays a critical role in regulating skeletal mineral metabolism during lactation. *Endocrinology*, *147*(9), 4010–4021. doi:10.1210/en.2005-1616 PMID:16675524

Working Group on Fortification of Salt with Iron. (1982). Use of Common Salt Fortified with Iron in the control and Prevention of Anaemia- A collaborative Study. *The American Journal of Clinical Nutrition*, *35*, 1442. doi:10.1093/ajcn/35.6.1442

World Health Organization. (1985). *Energy and Protein Requirements* (WHO Technical Report Series No. 724). WHO.

World Health Organization. (2003). *Global Vaccine Safety. Influenza vaccination of women during pregnancy*. Available from: https://www.who.int/vaccine_safety/committee/topics/in.uenza/pregnancy/Dec_2003/en/

World Health Organization. (2014). *Media centre. Hepatitis. A Fact sheet N 328*. Available from: http://www.who.int/mediacentre/factsheets/ fs328/en/

World Health Organization. (2015). *Expanded programme on immunization. Tetanus Neonatal Tetanus (NT)*. Available from: http://www.wpro.who.int/immunization/factsheets/tetanus_nt/en/

Chapter 4
High-Risk Pregnancies

ABSTRACT

Infant and child survival and their growth and development cannot be improved without good maternity care. Proper planning of births is a basic ingredient of any child survival package. Sexually transmitted diseases (STDs), and in particular HIV infections, unless adequately controlled, can impede further progress in child survival. There are great risks of neglecting sexual and reproductive health; a painful or detrimental transition from adolescence to adulthood can lead to ill effects in the long run. Early pregnancy/motherhood can be physically hazardous for girls and can jeopardize their educational attainment as well as economic potential. In particular, adolescent girls are vulnerable to HIV exposure and sexually transmitted infections (STIs), sexual coercion, violence, as well as exploitation. These have an enormous impact on the physical and mental health of an individual and have long-term implications for them, their offspring, their families, and their communities.

KEY FACTS

- Worldwide, eleven percent of all births and 14 percent of maternal deaths take place among 15 to 19 years old adolescents and 95 percent of adolescent births occur in the developing world (Patton et al, 2009; WHO, 2011).
- Adolescents are more susceptible to unintended pregnancies; every year 7.4 million (Guttmacher Institute, 2010) and 3 million (WHO,

DOI: 10.4018/978-1-7998-4357-3.ch004

2011) girls experience unintended pregnancies and unsafe abortions respectively.

- Globally, young people account for 41 percent of new infections among those, aged 15 years or older (UNAIDS, 2010).
- An estimated 1,300,000 adolescent girls are living with Human Immunodeficiency Virus (HIV) worldwide (UNICEF, 2011).
- Adolescents with disabilities are particularly vulnerable to sexual abuse and resultant unplanned pregnancies and HIV and other sexually transmitted infections (UNICEF, 2011).

INTRODUCTION

Maternity is a unique privilege for the mother but a unique burden on women's health. Though in some other aspects of reproductive health, the responsibility for child-bearing is shared by men and women yet the burden is heavily on women for both biological and social reasons. This relates to the burden of sexually transmitted diseases, the regulation of fertility as well as infertility (Fathalla and Fathalla, 2017).

Regulation of fertility is a key element of any strategizing motherhood. It decreases the number of unwanted pregnancies with a consequent decrease in total risk exposure as well as a decline in the number of unsafe abortions. Proper birth planning can also reduce the incidence as well as the number of high-risk pregnancies (Fathalla and Fathalla, 2017).

Globally, it is estimated that more than 220 million women in low middle-income countries (LMIC's) have an unmet need for family planning (Singh and Darroch, 2012). Overall, there has been little progress in increasing the use of contraception. While an increase in usage of contraception has been slightly higher among young adolescents as compared to older women, this group is more affected by failure of contraception. Moreover, the discontinuation rates and also the use of traditional methods of contraception are still noticed (Blanc et al, 2009; IPPF, 2010).

Estimates indicate that in developing countries, around 214 million women of reproductive age intending to want to avoid unwanted pregnancy; do not employ a modern method of contraception. Some methods of family planning help preventing HIV transmission and other sexually transmitted infections. The need for abortion, especially unsafe abortion, is reduced by

Family planning / contraception. Family planning strengthens the rights of the people to determine their children's number and maintain adequate spacing among them. Family planning / contraception reduce the incidence of higher-risk pregnancies and decreases maternal and infant mortality rates by preventing unintended pregnancy (WHO, 2018).

High-Risk Pregnancy

Bearing a baby is an act of creation. Pregnancy is much more than creating a new life; it is creating a new family. A baby, as a catalyst, creates news possibilities for more intimate relationship as well as new stresses in the closest relationships of woman with her partner, siblings and friends. For most women, pregnancy and new motherhood is a joy. But most mothers also experience worry, disappointment, guilt, competition, frustration, and even anger and fear (Sacks, 2017).

During pregnancy, some women experience some health issues or complications. These complications may affect the mother's own health, the health of the foetus or of both of them. Even women, who were apparently healthy before becoming pregnant, can suffer from various health related complications. Such complications make the pregnancy, a high-risk pregnancy.

Some disorders and conditions can mean that pregnancy is considered high-risk (about 6 to 8 percent of pregnancies in the United States of America) and in extreme cases may be contra-indicated. The gap in an access to adequate sexual and reproductive health care services represents a human rights violation that adversely affects millions of women worldwide, especially those living in low-and middle-income nations. Such a situation caused the pregnancy-associated deaths of 303,000 women during the year 2015. Of those dying women, 99 percent lived in low-and middle-income countries, where the probability of death from such causes is 30 times greater as compared to high-income countries (WHO, 2015). High-risk pregnancies are, thus, the focus of concern of the physicians specializing in maternal-fetal medicine (Guttmacher Institute, 2017).

There are various serious pre-existing disorders which may reduce the physical ability of a woman to survive her pregnancy. Such disorders include a wide range of congenital defects, i.e. the conditions with which the woman herself was born, diseases of the heart or reproductive organs etc. and/or the diseases acquired at any time during the woman's life.

General Risk Factors

There are numerous factors increasing the risk to the woman, the foetus/es or both of pregnancy complications beyond the normal level of risk. These factors may be present in a woman's medical profile either before she gets pregnant or any time during her pregnancy (US National Library of Medicine, 2013). These pre-existing factors may relate to her physical or mental health or to the social issues and/or a combination of those (Merck Sharp & Dohme, 2013).

Some common risk factors include the age of either parent at the time of pregnancy, which may be in continuum ranging from the adolescent parents to the older parents. Further, pregnancy over the age of 50 years may lead to complications of pregnancy.

There are some other risk factors, besides the age of mother, which are related to physical health of the mother. The higher incidences of pre-term birth and under-weight babies correlates with the pregnancy in women whose height is below 1.5 meters (5 feet), thus making it high risk pregnancy. The probable reason could be that such women are likely to have a small pelvis, thus resulting in such complications during childbirth as shoulder dystocia (Merck Sharp & Dohme, 2013).

Again, women with pre-pregnancy weight below 45.5 kilograms (100 pounds) are more prone to deliver underweight babies. On the other hand, obese women are more prone to produce very large babies, potentially leading to difficult childbirth. Besides, maternal obesity also raises the likelihood of developing gestational diabetes, high blood pressure, pre-eclampsia, experiencing post-term delivery and may also require a cesarean delivery (Merck Sharp & Dohme, 2013).

The inter-current diseases during pregnancy can also be the predisposing factors leading to complications of pregnancy. Any such disease or a condition that may not be necessarily caused directly by the pregnancy such as Diabetes Mellitus in pregnancy, Systemic Lupus Erythematosus (SLE) in pregnancy or thyroid disorder during pregnancy.

Other risk factors making any pregnancy a high risk pregnancy are an exposure to various environmental toxins during pregnancy or an exposure to recreational drugs in pregnancy like Ethanol consumption during pregnancy may cause foetal alcohol syndrome or foetal alcohol spectrum disorder. Exposure to some pharmaceutical drugs in pregnancy may contribute to other complications (Merck Sharp & Dohme, 2013). Anti-depressants, for example, may increase the risks of such outcomes as preterm delivery (Gavin, 2009).

A teratogen is anything that can contribute or increase the risk of developing a newborn with birth defect. These are the substances to which a mother is exposed to during her pregnancy. Teratogens include certain medicinal products, street drugs, alcohol, tobacco, toxic chemicals, some viruses and bacteria and certain other health conditions, such as uncontrolled diabetes. Teratogens may affect various body parts of the baby as they form as a baby grows in the womb. The neural tube, for example, closes during the first 3 to 5 weeks of pregnancy. During this period, teratogens may cause defects in the neural tube, such as Spina Bifida. During the whole pregnancy, certain organs are sensitive to teratogens. This covers the brain and spinal cord of the baby. Alcohol intake at any time during pregnancy adversely affects the brain and spinal cord of the baby (Stanford Children Health, 2020).

Tobacco smoking and pregnancy, when combined, cause twice the risk of premature rupture of membranes, placental abruption and placenta previa (Centers for Disease Control and Prevention, 2007). A host of negative outcomes for an infant and child, including low birth weight, preterm birth and various congenital defects have been related to the maternal tobacco use during pregnancy (Drake, et al, 2018). Cocaine exposure during pregnancy is also linked to, for example, premature birth, congenital defects and Attention Deficit Hyperactivity Disorder (ADHD) in children.

An exposure to methamphetamine during pregnancy can result in premature birth and congenital abnormalities (North Dakota Department of Health, 2011). Also, prenatal methamphetamine use is believed to have long-term effects in terms of brain development of child which may last for many years (North Dakota Department of Health, 2011). Other investigations have also revealed the short-term neonatal outcomes to include small deficits in infant neuro-behavioral functions and growth restriction, when compared to the control group of infants (Della Grotta, 2010). Cannabis use in pregnancy is also possibly associated with its adverse effects on the child development later in life.

However, there are certain other risks factors arising from the previous pregnancies. If there are complications experienced during a previous pregnancy, chances of complications are more likely to reoccur. There is an increased risk of very rapid labour and an excessive bleeding following delivery among women with a history of five previous pregnancies. Moreover, women with more than one foetus in her previous pregnancy suffer a higher risk of mislocated placenta (Merck Sharp & Dohme, 2013). Again, having more than one foetus in a single pregnancy is also associated with a likely risk of pregnancy.

Besides these biological and environmental factors, there are social and socio-economic factors contributing to the complications of pregnancy. In general, unmarried women and those in lower socio-economic groups are exposed to a higher risk of pregnancy, at least in part, due to the lack of adequate prenatal care (Merck Sharp & Dohme, 2013). In addition, pregnancies, which are unintended, prevent preconception care and delay prenatal care. They also preclude other preventive care, can disrupt life plans and, on an average, result in poorer physical and psychological results for the mother and for the offspring, if birth occurs (Eisenberg and Brown, 1995; Family Planning-Healthy People, 2020).

Fertility Regulation

Among many cultures, men are believed to have the right to control the childbearing of their wives. Thus, in many countries, when a woman wants to undergo sterilization, the law requires the consent of a husband. There is likelihood that with higher levels of education, couples communicate effectively on family planning and contraception use for keeping their family size and small adequate spacing among children. Also, more and more men adopt new models of masculinity, including being a responsible, caring husband and father (UNFPA, 2000).

The revolution leading to modern contraceptive technology rendered women the reliable birth control methods which can be used regardless of the male partner's need for cooperation. It was at a price. They had to take on the inconveniences and the involved risks. The male partner's role and responsibility dwindled when contraception was considered the business of a woman.

Therefore, women assume a disproportionate responsibility for contraception when compared to men. In the regulation of fertility, not only do women have an undue burden of responsibility but the methods available to women for use are those associated with potential health hazards. With the emergence of the Acquired Immune Deficiency Syndrome (AIDS) pandemic and the increasing prevalence of Sexually Transmitted Infections (STIs), where condom use is the only effective protection strategy other than abstinence, the importance of male involvement and responsibility has become much more important.

Various methods used for birth control can be broadly classified into barrier methods which prevent sperm cells from reaching the egg, methods preventing ovulation such as the birth control pills and other methods which allow fertilization of the egg and sperm but prevent implantation of the fertilized egg inside the uterus (womb) such as the IUD (intrauterine device). Besides, there are various other contraceptive methods which include injectables, diaphragms, cervical caps, spermicides and so on. There are non-supply methods also which include periodic abstinence or rhythm, withdrawal, douche, total sexual abstinence if practiced for contraceptive reasons, folk methods and many other methods (Stoppler, 2020).

The female partner's investigation of infertility is very elaborate and involves greater discomfort and risk. The treatment's burden falls heavily on the female partner as well. The promise of successful management, even for male infertility, is now shifting to assisted conception technologies where the major burden is assumed by the female partner.

In most societies, the psychological and social burden of infertility is far heavier on the woman. The status of a woman is often identified with her fertility and the failure to bear children is viewed as a cause for social disgrace or divorce. The infertile woman's suffering can be really real (UNFPA, 2000).

Unwanted Pregnancy

In every country, many women i.e. over half in some countries report unwanted pregnancy or mistimed their last pregnancy or child. There have been many negative repercussions of unwanted pregnancies and births for the children themselves, their siblings, their parents and the whole society. Older women and women with several children are faced with a higher risk of complications and death during childbirth, particularly in conditions of deprivation and where health care services are not sufficient.

Every year, more than one in four pregnancies worldwide end in abortions, many occurring under clandestine and unsafe conditions. Worldwide, unsafe abortion is a major contributing factor of maternal death. Moreover, it has a devastating effect on public health which is assessed by deaths, diseases, injuries and emergency care costs. More than half of women who seek abortion are married with children. Although in many countries, the proportion of young, unmarried women who have abortions is increasing. In order to reduce the number of abortions and the number of women dying as a result of unsafe abortions, there is a need to expand family planning services. This is particularly true when greater access to contraception and effective sexuality education are combined together (Population Action International, 1993).

Short Birth Intervals and Infant Mortality

Birth spacing offers significant advantages for both mothers and infants alike. Infants born less than one year after the last pregnancy of their mothers are far more likely to be undernourished and die than those born after a longer interval. Even after the first year of life, the risk of death posed by short birth intervals continues (UNFPA, 2000).

In addition, the older child's health may also be compromised when two children are born very close together. The term "kwashiorkor" is the type of malnutrition that is often seen when a child is weaned from the breast-milk too early as the mother is again pregnant. Due to too early weaning, children are considerably more susceptible to the vicious cycle of malnutrition and infection, often leading to death (UNFPA, 2000).

The higher infant mortality rates among infants who are closely-spaced may be partly due to the inadequate time for the body of mother to fully recover after her last pregnancy, which is called the "maternal depletion syndrome". This may be particularly true for those women who breastfeed their children for longer duration and among women, who are themselves malnourished and undergo heavy physical activities (UNFPA, 2000).

Infertility

Responsibility for infertility is commonly shared by the couple. An analysis of data compiled in a large multinational study by the World Health Organization revealed that only 12.8 percent of cases diagnosed a major factor in the female with no demonstrable cause in the male and only 7.5 percent of cases diagnosed a major factor in the male with no demonstrable cause in the female (World Health Organization, 1987). However, the burden of infertility is unequally shared for both biological and social reasons.

Pelvic infections, for example, account for about one-third of all infertility cases throughout the world and the percentage is much in Sub-saharan Africa (World Health Organization, 1987). The resultant infertility is also very difficult to treat. The infertility problem's magnitude cannot be ameliorated, except by a struggle of sexually transmitted diseases (STD's), by safer births which avoid postpartum infections and by decreasing its necessity or to resort to unsafe abortion practices.

Sexual Health, STDs and HIV/AIDS

In a marriage and for holding a family together, good sexual health and a healthy sexual relationship are very crucial. Sexually transmitted diseases (STDs), including HIV / AIDS, unfortunately have become an increasingly common threat to a healthy marriage. The extra-marital relationships of a husband carry the risk of not only becoming infected himself but also of bringing the infection to home which could kill his wife. The opposite is true too, though less often.

Sexually-Transmitted Diseases

HIV / AIDS has grown as a global pandemic that does not recognize national boundaries and poses great threats that many countries have yet to recognize. The pandemic is a deeply destabilizing force, which destroys the families and communities, seeding widespread misery and tragedy, thus decelerating the developmental prospects of the whole nations (UNFPA, 2000).

According to a study undertaken by the World Bank on the quantification of disease burden, Sexually Transmitted Diseases (STDs) are the second major cause of disease burden for young adult women in developing countries, thus accounts for 8.9 percent of the total disease burden in that age group (World Bank 1993). STD's are not amongst the first ten causes in males of the same age group and account only for 1.5 percent of the disease burden in adult men (World Bank, 1993).

For a blend of biological and social reasons, women are at a higher risk to get infected, are less likely to get care, are more difficult to get diagnosed, are more prone for severe disease sequelae and are also more subjected to social discrimination and its resulting consequences. Moreover, men have the control over the most effective method available for protection against STD's i.e. the condom. There does not exist even a simple and effective method of protection which a woman can use without her partner's cooperation.

Globally, it has been estimated that young women constitute more than 60 percent of all young people who live with HIV. This rate rises to 72 percent in Sub-Saharan Africa (UNICEF, 2011), with its prevalence among adolescent girls five times higher as compared to adolescent boys in some countries (UNICEF, 2014). The rate of STI's also indicates the highest prevalence among 20 to 24 year olds which is followed by 15 to 19 year olds, again with adolescent girls often bearing the higher burden (Dehne and Riedner, 2005).

Currently, it is estimated that 33.6 million people are infected with HIV/AIDS. In the year 1999, about 5.6 million people became newly infected with HIV/AIDS (UNAIDS, 1999c). More than 90 percent of these newly infected cases are present in developing countries where most common mode of transmission of HIV is through hetero-sexual transmission (The Population Council, 1999).

Young people are, currently, the group which is most severely impacted by HIV/AIDS. In the year 2009, young people, aged 15 and 24 years, accounted for 41 percent of all newly HIV infected adults. Worldwide, it has been estimated that there are five million young people, aged 15 to 25 years who are living with HIV infections. Later in the year 2016, 2.1 million people, aged 10 to 19 years, were found to be living with HIV and 2.6 lakh became newly infected with the virus. The number of adolescents living with HIV has risen by 30 percent between the years 2005 and 2016. Most of these young people live in Sub-Saharan Africa where most young women are up to 8 times more vulnerable to HIV as compared to young men (UNAID, 2015).

Biologically, the immature reproductive and immune systems of adolescent girls translate to their increased susceptibility to STI's and HIV transmission (UNICEF, 2014). In addition to biological vulnerability, cultural and socioeconomic factors, particularly social inequality and exclusion, as well as having older partners, increase their susceptibility to infection.

The presence of other sexually transmitted infections, especially ulcerative infections, facilitates the transmission of HIV infection. It has been found that every year; there are 12 million new cases of syphilis, 89 million of chlamydia, 62 million of gonorrhoea and 170 million of trichomoniasis. In these cases, too, women are at higher risk of infection (The Population Council, 1999).

Men are twice as likely to get their partners infected as women. Biologically also, females are more vulnerable to infection. Moreover, many women do not understand the nature of transmission of STD / HIV and many are in denial about the extramarital sexual activity of their husband. Finally, most women do not have the say to deny their husbands or partners for sexual activity or to insist them to use a contraceptive.

Treatment of STI's is important because this can facilitate the transmission of HIV as well as cause long lasting damage. An access to any acceptable and affordable STI/HIV services is available to only a minority of adolescents. Moreover, comprehensive and accurate knowledge about HIV is very low as well as HIV testing in this age group is rare in most of the countries (Idele et al, 2014).

Young people with HIV have poor outcomes; while an analysis of a study carried out between the years 2005 and 2012 estimated a 32 percent decrease in AIDS-related deaths among non-adolescents (aged 0 to 9 years and aged 20 and older), there was a 50 percent increase in AIDS-related deaths among adolescents (aged 10 to 19 years), especially among boys (Leach-Lemens, 2014).

Mother-to-Child Transmission of HIV/AIDS and Other STD's

The early life chances of survival are even grimmer for children whose mothers are infected with HIV because mother-to child transmission is the greatest source of HIV infection among children below the age of 15 years. AIDS is now the biggest single cause of death among children in a growing number of countries. In Southern Africa urban centers, HIV rates of 20 to 30 percent among pregnant women tested at antenatal clinics is common (UNAIDS, 1999a).

In the year 1998, of all those newly infected HIV cases, 10 percent were children, the vast majority of whom acquired the virus from their mothers. The virus may transmit during pregnancy, infancy or breastfeeding. Africa is an abode of 90 percent of the world's children who are infected with HIV. This could be possibly due to very high incidence of female HIV infection along with their high fertility rates. However, there appears to be a rapid rise in the number of HIV-infected children in India and South East Asia where there are no preventive measures being undertaken. In industrialized countries, the risk of a baby acquiring the virus from an infected mother ranges from 15 to 25 percent and in the developing countries; it ranges from 25 to 45 percent. It was estimated that nearly 4.5 million children below 15 years, have been infected with HIV and more than 3 million of these children have already died of AIDS. AIDS, thus, is a threat to reverse the period of uniform progress in child survival which is achieved through such measures as the promotion of breastfeeding, immunization and oral rehydration etc. (UNAIDS, 1999a).

The Joint United Nations Program on HIV / AIDS (UNAIDS) projects that AIDS may have caused a raised mortality among children under 5 years of age by more than 100 percent in regions which are most affected by the virus by the year 2010 (UNAIDS, 1999a). Congenital and perinatal sexually transmitted infections also have grave long-term consequences. Syphilis, for example, leads to blindness, deafness, paralysis, bone illness and gonorrhoea.

A new drug, called nevirapine (Viramune), offers some hope to resource-poor countries. An anti-retroviral drug, nevirapine, that slows down the reproduction of HIV, has been reported to bring down the infection to half and is cheaper than other drugs. Nevirapine has also received the clearance from U.S. Food and Drug Administration for treatment of paediatric HIV/AIDS and is used to treat HIV-positive pregnant women in Uganda (now a leader in HIV/AIDS control efforts) (UNAIDS, 1999b).

Barriers and Challenges

Evidence from international literature suggests that interventions that focus exclusively on individual motivation and behaviour change are only partially effective. In general, female volunteers have less control over their choice to get engaged in high-risk behaviours. Socio-cultural factors have a significant influence on their risk behaviors as well as on their access to reproductive health services. In the global literature, though the association between socio-cultural factors and sexual and reproductive health is well recognized but has received little attention. An insight on these factors is needed so that the government and other healthcare providers can better understand and address the needs of this vulnerable population (UNFPA, 2011).

Socio-cultural factors have a significant influence on the female population's sexual and reproductive health behaviour as well as on their access to health services. There is a need to properly understand the norms and positive values derived from or influenced by religious and cultural traditions so as to use them as creative instruments to create awareness among particularly vulnerable women of sexual and reproductive health (UNFPA, 2011).

Little literature is available on the association between socio-cultural factors and female population's sexual and reproductive health although some research has been undertaken to study the impact of socio-cultural factors on sexual and reproductive health in general and among rural women in particular. It has been observed that health or basic education, gender differences in roles and responsibilities as well as cultural values do persist and create patterns of inequality in education, labour and decision-making power though gender-related issues may not reveal extreme forms of inequality in life expectancy. Though the principle of gender equality is promoted by the constitutional and legal provisions and to prevent females from participating in political, economic, cultural and social activities is considered a criminal offence but society is still dominated by men and women have yet to take full advantage of their rights (UNFPA, 2011).

Given that most female adolescents are young, reproductive health care services are needed by them. Yet this need of reproductive health care services has been recognized and addressed by very few programs or interventions. It has been revealed through the literature available that young female adolescents had little knowledge of STIs, HIV and AIDS. They had to recourse to self-medication instead of seeking support at a health facility. Moreover, they had a significantly lower rate of use of contraception in comparison to their older counterparts. It was also reported that the frequency of health risk behavior regarding sexual and reproductive health was higher among young adolescents. However, a United Nations Report in 2010 attributed this higher frequency of health risk behavior regarding sexual and reproductive health not only to the behavioral and situational factors but also to lack of access to various government health services. It was also found that most of the government interventions, such as media information, behaviour change communication and other information and education activities were often ineffective in reaching female adolescents for the prevention of HIV (UNFPA, 2011).

Hence, the issues of health system problems related to access, availability, affordability, acceptability, equity and quality, policy practice or health care delivery problems need to be addressed on priority basis so as to achieve the targets of millennium development goals.

REFERENCES

Blanc, A. K., Tsui, A. O., Croft, T. N., & Trevitt, J. L. (2009). Patterns and trends in adolescents' contraceptive use and discontinuation in developing countries and comparisons with adult women. *International Perspectives on Sexual and Reproductive Health, 35*(2), 63–71. doi:10.1363/3506309 PMID:19620090

Centers for Disease Control and Prevention. (2007). *Preventing Smoking and Exposure to Secondhand Smoke Before, During, and After Pregnancy Archived 2011-09-11 at the Wayback Machine*. Author.

Centers for Disease Control and Prevention. (2009). *Tobacco Use and Pregnancy: Home*. Author.

Dehne, K., & Riedner, G. (2005). *Sexually Transmitted Infections among adolescents: The need for adequate health services*. WHO.

Della Grotta, S., LaGasse, L. L., Arria, A. M., Derauf, C., Grant, P., Smith, L. M., Shah, R., Huestis, M., Liu, J., & Lester, B. M. (2010). Patterns of methamphetamine use during pregnancy: Results from the Infant Development, Environment, and Lifestyle (IDEAL) Study. *Maternal and Child Health Journal, 14*(4), 519–527. doi:10.100710995-009-0491-0 PMID:19565330

Eisenberg, L. & Brown, S.H. (1995). *The best intentions: unintended pregnancy and the well-being of children and families*. Washington, DC: National Academy Press.

Family planning- Healthy People (2020). Archived from the original on 2010-12-28. Retrieved 2011-08-18.

Fathalla, M.F. (1999). *Health and Being a Woman*. Figo.org/sites/default/files/uploads/PublicationsandResourcesFathallahfiles/A/4%20Health%20and%20being%20a%20woman.pdf.

Fathalla, M. F., & Fathalla, M. M. (2017). Sexual and Reproductive Health: Overview. International Encyclopedia of Public Health, 5, 481-490.

Gavin, A. R., Holzman, C., Siefert, K., & Tian, Y. (2009). Maternal depressive symptoms, depression, and psychiatric medication use in relation to risk of preterm delivery. *Women's Health Issues, 19*(5), 325–334. doi:10.1016/j.whi.2009.05.004 PMID:19733802

Guttmacher Institute. (2010). *Facts on the Sexual and Reproductive Health of Adolescent Women in the Developing World*. International Planned Parenthood Federation.

Guttmacher Institute. (2017). *Unintended Pregnancy in the United States*. www.guttmacher.org

Idele, P., Gillespie, A., Porth, T., Suzuki, C., Mahy, M., Kasedde, S., & Luo, C. (2014). Epidemiology of HIV and AIDS among adolescents: Current status, inequities, and data gaps. *Journal of Acquired Immune Deficiency Syndromes, 66*(2), S144–S153. doi:10.1097/QAI.0000000000000176 PMID:24918590

International Federation of Gynecology and Obstetrics. (2011). *Adolescent sexual and reproductive health (ASRH)*. London: FIGO. Retrieved from https://www.go.org/.go-projectpublications

International Planned Parenthood Federation. (2010). *Facts on the sexual and reproductive health of adolescent women in the developing world.* New York: Guttmacher Institute. Retrieved from https://www.guttmacher.org/pubs/FB-Adolescents-SRH.pdf

Leach-Lemens, C. (2014). *Adolescent deaths from AIDS rising, especially among boys.* London: National Academy of Medicine (NAM) Publications. http://www.aidsmap.com/Adolescent-deaths-from-AIDS rising-especially-among-boys/page/2893246/

Merck Sharp & Dohme. (2013). Risk factors present before pregnancy. In *Merck Manual Home Health Handbook.* Author.

Norris, S. A., Osmond, C., Gigante, D., Kuzawa, C. W., Ramakrishnan, L., Lee, N. R., Ramirez-Zea, M., Richter, L. M., Stein, A. D., Tandon, N., & Fall, C. H. D. (2012). Size at birth, weight gain in infancy and childhood, and adult diabetes risk in five low- or middle-income country birth cohorts. *Diabetes Care, 35*(1), 72–79. doi:10.2337/dc11-0456 PMID:22100968

North Dakota Department of Health. (2011). *New mother fact sheet: methamphetamine use during pregnancy.* Author.

Patrick Drake, M. S., Driscoll, A. K., & Mathews, M. S. (2018). *Cigarette Smoking During Pregnancy.* National Centre for Health Statistics.

Patton, G. C., Coffey, C., Sawyer, S. M., Viner, R. M., Haller, D. M., Bose, K., Vos, T., Ferguson, J., & Mathers, C. D. (2009). Global patterns of mortality in young people: A systematic analysis of population health data. *Lancet, 374*(9693), 881–892. doi:10.1016/S0140-6736(09)60741-8 PMID:19748397

Population Action International. (1993). *Expanding Access to Safe Abortion: Key Policy Issues.* Author.

Sacks, A. (2017). *The birth of a mother.* Retrieved from https://www.nytimes.com/2017/05/08/well/family/the-birth-of-a-mother.html

Singh, S., & Darroch, J. E. (2012). *Adding it up: Costs and benefits of contraceptive service. Estimates for 2012.* New York: Guttmacher Institute and UNFPA. Retrieved from http://www. guttmacher.org/pubs/AIU-2012-estimates.pdf

Stanford Children Health. (2020). *Medical Genetics: Teratogens.* Retrieved from https://www.stanfordchildrens.org/en/topic/default?id=teratogens-overview-90-P09519

Stoppler, M. C. (2020). *15 Birth control options (Types and Side effects).* Retrieved from https://www.medicinenet.com/birth_control_methods/article.htm

The Population Council. (1999). Sexually Transmitted Infections. In *Reproductive Tract Infections: A Set of Factsheets*. The Population Council.

UNAID. (2015). *Young People, HIV and AIDS*. Global Information and Education on HIV and AIDS.

UNAIDS. (1999a). *Questions and answers: Mother-to-Child Transmission (MTCT) of HIV: Background Briefing*. UNAIDS.

UNAIDS. (1999b). *Technical Working Group Meeting to Review New Research Findings for the Prevention of Mother-to-Child Transmission of HIV*. UNAIDS.

UNAIDS. (1999c). *AIDS Epidemic Update: December1999*. UNAIDS.

UNAIDS. (2010). *Global Report: UNAIDS Report on the Global AIDS Epidemic, Joint United Nations Programme on HIV/AIDS*. UNAIDS.

UNFPA. (2000). *Women Empowerment and Reproductive Health: Links throughout the Life Cycle*. United Nations Population Fund.

UNFPA. (2011). *Socio-cultural influences on the reproductive health of migrant women.* Retrieved from https://www.unfpa.org/sites/default/files/pub-pdf/Migrant_Vietnam_.pdf

UNICEF. (2011). *Opportunity in crises: Preventing HIV from early adolescence to early childhood.* United Nations Children's Fund.

UNICEF. (2014). *Goal: Promote gender equality and empower women*. http://www.unicef. org/mdg/index_genderequality.htm

US National Library of Medicine (2013). Health problems in pregnancy. *Medline Plus*.

Viner, R. M., Coffey, C., Mathers, C., Bloem, P., Costello, A., Santelli, J., & Patton, G. C. (2011). 50-Year mortality trends in children and young people: A study of 50 low-income, middle-income, and high income countries. *Lancet*, *377*(9772), 1162–1174. doi:10.1016/S0140-6736(11)60106-2 PMID:21450338

World Bank. (1993). *World Development Report- Investing in Health.* Oxford University Press.

World Health Organization. (2011a). *Preventing early pregnancy and poor reproductive outcomes among adolescents in developing countries.* World Health Organization.

World Health Organization. (2011b). *Mortality estimates by cause, age, and sex for the year 2008.* World Health Organization.

World Health Organization. (2015). Trends in maternal mortality: 1990 to 2015: Estimates by WHO, UNICEF, UNFPA. World Bank Group and the United Nations Population Division.

World Health Organization. (2018). *Family planning/Contraception.* Retrieved from https://www.who.int/news-room/fact-sheets/detail/family-planning-contraception

Chapter 5
Complications of Pregnancy

ABSTRACT

Although the majority of pregnancies are uneventful, sometimes complications do happen. Pregnancy complications are the conditions or pathological processes associated with pregnancy. They can occur during or after pregnancy and range from minor discomforts to serious diseases that require medical interventions. They can involve the mother's health, the baby's health, or both. Complication of pregnancy can cause maternal morbidity and mortality. The most common causes of maternal mortality are maternal bleeding, maternal sepsis, hypertensive disease, obstructed labour, and pregnancy with the consequence of abortion, which includes miscarriage, ectopic pregnancy, and medical abortion. The primary means of preventing maternal deaths is to provide rapid access to emergency obstetric care, including treatment of haemorrhage, infection, hypertension, and obstructed labour. Proper antenatal care can reduce the maternal mortality rate by reducing the number of pregnancies among women of reproductive age. Thus, adequate monitoring and appropriate intervention strategies should be provided for better maternal and fetal outcome.

KEY FACTS

- Half a million women die each year due to complications of pregnancy and childbirth; 99 percent of these deaths occur in developing countries (WHO, 2014).

DOI: 10.4018/978-1-7998-4357-3.ch005

- Impaired foetal growth is more common in pregnancies occurring before the age of 18 years and low birth weight is an important risk factor for adult onset of diabetes (Norris, 2012).
- Though mortality among 1 to 4-year old declined by more than 80 percent over the past five decades whereas adolescent mortality rates only improved by 41 to 48 percent (Viner et al, 2011).
- In the United States, severe complications of pregnancy, childbirth and puerperium affect 1.6 percent mothers (CDC, 2015) and 1.5 percent of mothers in Canada (The Society of Obstetricians and Gynecologists of Canada (SOGC), 2009).

INTRODUCTION

Majority of pregnancies normally take place without any complications. Some pregnant women, however, will experience complications that can affect their health, the health of their baby or both. Diseases or conditions that the mother had before becoming pregnant can sometimes lead to complications during pregnancy. There can be some complications during delivery. Even with complications, early detection and prenatal care may reduce any additional risks to both mother and child.

There is, however, no clear distinction between the symptoms and discomforts of pregnancy and the complications of pregnancy. Though the symptoms of normal pregnancy do not generally interfere with the routine activities of mother in her day to day life or do not pose any risk to her health or that of her baby yet in other cases, similar symptoms may manifest either as discomfort or as complications, which usually depend on the severity of those symptoms. For instance, mild nausea is only a discomfort as morning sickness but if severe and accompanied by vomiting, it may cause an imbalance of water and electrolytes and then it can be classified as a complication of pregnancy (hyperemesis gravidarum).

Complications of pregnancy are, therefore, the health related issues which are caused due to pregnancy. Complications which occur primarily during delivery are termed **obstetric labour complications** and complications that occur primarily after birth of the child are called **puerperal disorders**. Any difficulty or abnormality that arises during the process of labour or the delivery is called obstetric labour complication.

The Trust for America's Health (TAH) reported about one-third of American births had some complications as of 2011, many of which were directly related to the health of the mother, including rising rates of obesity, type 2 diabetes and physical inactivity. In an effort to reduce neonatal and maternal death rates, the U.S. Centers for Disease Control and Prevention (CDC) has led an initiative to improve women's health prior to conception (Levi et al, 2011).

In the United States, severe complications of pregnancy, childbirth and puerperium affect 1.6 percent mothers (CDC, 2015) and 1.5 percent of mothers in Canada (The Society of Obstetricians and Gynecologists of Canada (SOGC), 2009).

Globally, the complications related to pregnancy, childbirth and puerperium declined from 377,000 deaths in the year 1990 to 230,600 deaths in the year 2016. Maternal bleeding, maternal sepsis and other infections, pregnancy induced hypertension, obstructed labor and pregnancy ending in abortion which includes miscarriage, ectopic pregnancy and elective abortion were reported to be the most common causes of maternal mortality (GBD, 2016).

Multiple Pregnancies

A multiple pregnancy is the culmination of a single pregnancy in which a mother gives birth to two or more off-springs. This term is commonly pertinent to placental species. Multiple births take place with varying frequencies in most of the mammals. Multiple births are usually named as per the number of offspring such as twins, triplets and so on. Multiple births are exceptionally rare in the largest mammals and are an exception in human species as well.

A multiple pregnancy occurs as a result of either a single egg undergoing fertilization which splits to produce identical fetuses or as a result of the fertilization of multiple eggs to produce fraternal fetuses or as a combination of two. A multiple pregnancy resulting from a single zygote (fertilized egg) is termed as monozygotic, is termed as dizygotic from two zygotes and is termed as polyzygotic from three or more zygotes. Similarly, the siblings from a multiple birth are termed as monozygous, if identical or polyzygous, if fraternal (NICE, 2011).

Each fertilized egg, called zygote, grows in to a single embryo or may split into two or more each having same genetic material. Foetuses developing from different zygotes are fraternal which share only half of the genetic material, as normal full birth siblings do. Foetuses that result from the same zygote share 100 percent of the genetic material and are thus identical. Except for Klinefelter syndrome (also known as XXY syndrome and 47 XXY syndromes), identical twins always have the same sex (NICE, 2011).

Multiple pregnancies are also classified according to how one or more placentas and amniotic sacs surround the foetuses; the placentas are referred to as "chorions" (NICE, 2011). One placenta is shared by monochorionic foetuses; dichorionic twins, trichorionic triplets etc. having a separate placenta in each. One amniotic sac is shared by monoamniotic foetuses; diamniotic twins each have their own bag, as are triamniotic triplets, etc. There are many possible combinations with dichorionic triamniotic triplets, for example, one fetus has a separate placenta and two of the fetuses share a placenta and each has its own amniotic sac.

Etiology

Multiple births among humans may occur either naturally (the woman naturally ovulates multiple eggs or the fertilized egg splits into two) or as an outcome of infertility treatments such as IVF (in-vitro fertilization) where in order to compensate for the lower quality or fertility drugs, several embryos are often transferred which can cause multiple eggs to mature in one ovulatory cycle.

There are several factors which seem to increase the possibility of woman naturally conceiving the multiple births. These factors include the age of mother i.e. women over 35 years of age are more prone to have multiple births as compared to their younger counterparts (ACOG, 2016). However, for reasons not yet known, the older a woman is, the more likely she is to have a multiple birth naturally. It is theorized that this is due to the higher level of Follicle-Stimulating Hormone (FSH) that older women sometimes have as their ovaries respond more slowly to Follicle-Stimulating Hormone (FSH) stimulation (Beemsterboer et al, 2006).

Again, mother's use of fertility drugs has the likelihood of multiple births. It is estimated that around 35 percent of pregnancies as an outcome of fertility treatments such as IVF (in-vitro fertilization) result in more than one child per pregnancy. The incidence of multiple births has become more frequent and hence more visible by the increasing use of fertility drugs and consequently leading to an increased rate of multiple births.

Risks Factors

Premature Birth

Babies born from multiple-birth pregnancies are much more likely to result in premature births than those from single pregnancies. It is estimated that 51 percent of twins and 91 percent of triplets are born preterm as compared to 9.4 percent in singletons (Alexander et al, 1998). Again, 14 percent of twins and 41 percent of triplets are even born very preterm as compared to 1.7 percent in singletons (Alexander et al, 1998).

As recently as until the year 2015, there was no way to stop twins from being born early (Yamasmit et al, 2015). In women with single pregnancies, drugs called betamimetics can relax the muscles of the uterus and delay childbirth (Neilson et al, 2014). Giving betamimetics helps giving more time to transfer the mother to a hospital with a special care unit and to give steroids for the baby's lung development (Neilson et al, 2014).

However, evidence is needed to support whether or not oral betamimetics be given to women with twin pregnancies to reduce the risk of preterm birth (Yamasmit et al, 2015). In some studies, the use of betamimetics has reduced the rate of preterm labour in twin pregnancies. However, the studies are too small to draw any solid conclusions (Yamasmit et al, 2015). Likewise, due to the small sample sizes in the studies, there has not been evidence to support the fact that putting a stitch in the neck of the womb (a cervical suture) will prevent premature birth in women carrying more than one baby (Rafael et al, 2014).

Low Birth Weight

The preterm births also result in multiple offsprings who have lower birth weight as compared to birth weight of singletons. The Kupresak triplets of Mississauga, Ontario, Canada had their combined weight at birth of 17 lbs, 2.7 ounces, set a world record in 2008, are an exception (Le, 2011).

Incomplete Separation

Multiples can be monochorionic i.e. sharing the same chorion, with the resulting threat of twin-to-twin transfusion syndrome. Such multiples can be monoamniotic, which share the common amniotic sac, leading to the risk of compression of the umbilical cord and of nuchal cord. Conjoined twins may exist in very rare cases, possibly impairing the functions of the bodies ' internal organs.

Mortality Rate (Stillbirth)

The mortality rate of multiples is also known to be higher. Multiple births are often stillborn while the risk for singletons is not as high as in case of multiple births.

A review of literature of multiple pregnancies reveals a study performed on one set of seven-folds and octuplets, two sets of sextuplets, eight sets of quintuplets, 17 sets of quadruplets and 228 sets of triplets. After undertaking this study, Hammond found that the mean gestational age (how many weeks when birthed) was 33.4 weeks for triplets and 31 weeks for quadruplets. Results revealed that that stillbirth often take place 3 to 5 weeks before the woman reaches full gestation period. It was also found that sextuplets or higher almost always end in the death of the foetuses (Hammond, 1998).

Although multiples are at an increased risk of born still, there is no conclusive evidence to support whether or not the actual mortality rate is higher in multiples than in singletons.

Hyperemesis Gravidarum

Hyperemesis gravidarum (HG) is a pregnancy complication characterized by severe nausea and vomiting, leading to weight loss, possibly resulting from dehydration. There may also be some feeling of faint. It's seen as severe form of morning sickness. However, symptoms usually recover after 20th week of gestation but may last for the whole duration of the pregnancy (Office on Women's Health, 2010).

Technically speaking, hyperemesis gravidarum is defined as the incidence of greater than three vomiting episodes daily so that there is weight loss of 5 percent or three kilograms and there is presence of ketones in the urine (Jueckstock et al, 2010). Other probable causes of symptoms, including urinary tract infection and an overactive thyroid gland, should be excluded (Sheehan, 2007).

Hyperemesis gravidarum is estimated to affect 0.3 to 2.0 percent of pregnant women (Goodwin, 2008). Previously, it was known as a common cause of death during pregnancy but now, with proper treatment, mortality due to this is very rare (Kumar, 2011; DeLegge, 2007). Those affected with hyperemesis gravidarum have a lesser risk of miscarriage but are more prone to preterm birth (Ferri, 2012). Due to severity of symptoms of hyperemesis gravidarum, some pregnant women prefer to undergo an abortion (Gabbe, 2012).

Hyperemesis gravidarum often occurs in the first trimester and continues significantly longer than the morning sickness (Ahmed et al, 2013). Though there is nearly complete relief from the symptoms of morning sickness near the beginning of their second trimester in some women while other women may experience severe symptoms until they give birth to their babies and some women may experience the symptoms even after giving birth. However, a small proportion of pregnant women rarely vomit but the feeling of nausea still impacts most though not all of the same concerns that hyperemesis with vomiting does.

Etiology

Vomiting is a common condition which affects about 50 percent of pregnant women with another 25 percent of pregnant women suffering from nausea (Niebyl, 2010). However, there is only 0.3 to1.5 percent incidence of hyperemesis gravidarum (Sheehan, 2007). After preterm labour, it is the second most common cause of hospitalization in first half of pregnancy (Summers, 2012).

Factors causing hyperemesis gravidarum include Helicobacter pylori caused infection, an increase in the production of thyroid hormone, young age; Pre-pregnancy less Body Mass Index (BMI), multiple pregnancies, molar pregnancies as well as past history of hyperemesis gravidarum are likely to be linked with the onset of hyperemesis gravidarum (Summers, 2012).

Risk Factors

The exact cause of hyperemesis gravidarum is not known (Jueckstock et al, 2010). However, various risk factors are first pregnancy, multiple pregnancy, obesity, prior or family history of hyperemesis gravidarum, trophoblastic disorder and a history of eating disorder (Jueckstock et al, 2010; Ferri, 2012). Diagnosis is usually made on the basis of the observed signs and symptoms of hyperemesis gravidarum (Jueckstock et al, 2010).

Signs and Symptoms

In case of severe vomiting, it may cause the loss of 5 percent or more of pre-pregnancy body weight of mother which is caused by the loss of water and electrolytes (Summers, 2012). Dehydration may occur, thus causing ketosis and constipation (Ahmed et al, 2013). Nutritional deficiency disorders may also occur such as deficiency of vitamin B_1 (thiamine), vitamin B_6 (pyridoxine) or vitamin B_{12} (cobalamin). An imbalance of metabolism may also occur such as metabolic ketoacidosis (Summers, 2012) or thyrotoxicosis (Matthews and Syed, 2011). Moreover, physical and emotional stress also takes place due to the difficulty in carrying out the activities of daily life.

Symptoms are, further, intensified with hunger, fatigue, antenatal vitamins and minerals, especially those containing iron and diet (Carlson et al, 2004). Many women with hyperemesis gravidarum are very sensitive to odours in their environment; certain odours may aggravate the symptoms of hyperemesis gravidarum. Another symptom experienced by some pregnant women is excessive salivation, also known as sialorrhea gravidarum.

Treatment

Treatment of hyperemesis gravidarum among pregnant women includes the Oral Rehydration Therapy (ORT) by drinking plenty of fluids and having a bland diet which comprise the first-line treatment (*Office on Women's Health, 2010*). Recommendations may also include electrolyte-replacement drinks, intake of B-vitamins such as thiamine and a high protein diet as per the severity of the condition of the pregnant women (*Jueckstock et al, 2010; Gabbe, 2012*).

Hyperemesis gravidarum is treated as an emergency due to its potential for severe dehydration and other complications. Some pregnant women with severe symptoms of hyperemesis gravidarum may require intravenous fluids (*Office on Women's Health, 2010*). With respect to medications, pyridoxine or metoclopramide are preferred *(Sheehan, 2007)*. Hospitalization may be required in extreme cases of hyperemesis gravidarum (*Jueckstock et al, 2010*). Psycho-therapy may improve the outcomes of the condition among pregnant women (*Jueckstock et al, 2010*).

However, women who do not respond to intravenous rehydration and medication, may need the supportive nutrition. Patients may be given parenteral nutrition (a PICC line for intravenous feeding) or enteral nutrition through a nasogastric tube or a nasojejunal tube. Limited evidence from trials is available to support supplementation with vitamin B6 for the improvement in the results (Matthews et al, 2015). A physician might also prescribe Vitamin B_1 and folic acid supplementation to prevent Wernicke's encephalopathy (Bourne et al, 2006). An oversupply of nutrition (hyperalimentation) may be required in some cases to maintain the volume requirements and allow for weight gain of the pregnant woman (Evans, 2007).

Complications of Hyperemesis Gravidarum

Pregnant Woman

In case if hyperemesis gravidarum is not adequately treated, malnutrition, hypoglycemia, anemia, hyponatremia, Wernicke's encephalopathy, kidney failure, coagulopathy, atrophy, jaundice, deep vein thrombosis, pulmonary embolism, splenic avulsion, vasospasms of cerebral arteries are the possible consequences for the pregnant woman (Summers, 2012). Depression and post-traumatic stress disorder (Christodoulou-Smith et al, 2011) are common secondary complications of hyperemesis gravidarum, for which the emotional support can be beneficial for the patients (Summers, 2012).

Infant

The effects of hyperemesis gravidarum on the foetus are mainly due to an electrolyte imbalance caused by hyperemesis gravidarum in the mother (Bourne et al, 2006). Moreover, infants born to mothers showing severe hyperemesis gravidarum, in whom weight gain is below 7 kilograms (15 lb) during pregnancy, are of low birth weight, smaller for their age of gestation and are born before 37 weeks of gestation (Ahmed et al, 2013).

In contrast, infants born to mothers with hyperemesis gravidarum, with weight gain of more than 7 kilograms during pregnancy, seem similar to infants who are born from uncomplicated pregnancies (Dodds et al, 2006). The rates of neonatal mortality in infants born to mothers with hyperemesis gravidarum as compared to infants who are born to mothers without hyperemesis gravidarum do not differ significantly (Summers, 2012). However, children born to mothers with under-treated hyperemesis gravidarum have a four-fold increase in neuro-behavioral diagnoses (Fejzo et al, 2015).

Gestational Diabetes Mellitus (GDM)

Gestational Diabetes Mellitus (GDM) is a condition in which a non-diabetic woman has high blood sugar level during pregnancy. Gestational Diabetes Mellitus (GDM) is carbohydrate intolerance resulting in hyperglycemia with its onset during pregnancy. Gestational Diabetes Mellitus often leads to few symptoms. However, it raises the risk of pre-eclampsia, depression and the delivery requiring a caesarean section in pregnant women (NIDDK, 2014).

Gestational Diabetes Mellitus (GDM) is formally defined as “a degree of glucose intolerance with its onset or first appearance in pregnancy” (Metzger and Coustan, 1998). The possibility that a woman may have previously undiagnosed diabetes mellitus or may develop diabetes coincidentally during pregnancy is acknowledged by the above definition. It is also irrelevant to the diagnosis whether the symptoms of diabetes diminish after pregnancy (American Diabetes Association, 2004). A woman is diagnosed with gestational diabetes when the glucose intolerance continues beyond 24 to 28 weeks of gestation.

Etiology

Gestational diabetes affects almost 3 to 9 percent of pregnancies depending on the population studied (Donovan and McIntyre, 2010). It is especially common during the third trimester i.e. last three months of pregnancy (NIDDK, 2014). It affects one percent of those under the age of 20 years and 13 percent of those above 44 years (Donovan and McIntyre, 2010).

A number of ethnic groups i.e. Asians, American Indians, Indigenous Australians, and Pacific Islanders are at a higher risk of developing diabetes mellitus (Donovan and McIntyre, 2010; NIDDK, 2014). In almost 90 percent of the cases, gestational diabetes mellitus resolves after the baby is born (NIDDK, 2014). However, pregnant women are at a higher risk of type 2 diabetes mellitus (Donovan and McIntyre, 2010).

Moreover, mothers with poorly treated gestational diabetes mellitus give birth to babies who are also at an enhanced risk of being too big, having low blood sugar level after birth and develop jaundice (NIDDK, 2014). It may also result in a stillbirth, if untreated (NIDDK, 2014). Later in life too, children have an increased risk to be overweight and also develop type 2 diabetes mellitus (NIDDK, 2014).

Risk Factors

Gestational diabetes is caused by not enough insulin being secreted in the setting of insulin resistance (NIDDK, 2014). Classical risk factors for developing gestational diabetes mellitus include overweight mother, previous history of gestational diabetes, a family history of type 2 diabetes and Polycystic Ovarian Syndrome (PCOD) (NIDDK, 2014).

Moreover, a previous diagnosis of gestational diabetes mellitus or pre-diabetes, impaired glucose tolerance or impaired fasting glycemia could be other risk factors. A family history revealing a first-degree relative with type 2 diabetes mellitus may contribute significantly to its occurrence. Other precipitating factors could be the maternal age and the paternal age. Risk to women increases with age (especially for women above 35 years of age). Results of a study revealed that a father over the age of 55 years was also at risk of developing Gestational diabetes mellitus (Khandwala et al, 2018).

Another risk factor could be the ethnicity i.e. African-Americans, Afro-Caribbeans, Native Americans, Hispanics, Pacific Islanders and people originating from South Asia are at higher risk. The risk for pregnant women increases by a factor of 2.1, 3.6 and 8.6 for overweight, obese or severely obese respectively (Chu et al, 2007).

A previous pregnancy with poor obstetric history which resulted in a child with a macrosomia (high birth weight >90th centile or >4000 gm (8 lbs 12.8 oz) can be another risk factor. Other genetic risk factors include at least 10 genes where certain polymorphism is associated with an increased risk of gestational diabetes mellitus, most notably TCF7L2 (Zhang et al, 2013).

In addition to the above risk factors, statistics show a double risk of Gestational Diabetes Mellitus (GDM) among smokers (Bjørge et al, 2004). Some studies have looked at more controversial potential risk factors, such as short stature (Ma et al, 2007). Polycystic Ovarian Syndrome (PCOD) is also a risk factor (Ross, 2006), although the relevant evidence remains controversial (Toulis et al, 2009).

Diagnosis

Diagnosis of Gestational Diabetes Mellitus is done by screening through blood tests (NIDDK, 2014). For pregnant women at a normal risk, screening is recommended between 24 and 28 weeks of gestation (NIDDK, 2014; Donovan and McIntyre, 2010). For pregnant women at high risk, testing may be done at the first prenatal visit (NIDDK, 2014). About 40 to 60 percent of women with Gestational Diabetes Mellitus have no demonstrable risk factor; for this reason, many advocate to screen all pregnant women, irrespective of their status (Precis, 1994).

Typically, pregnant women having Gestational Diabetes Mellitus show no symptoms which is another reason for universal screening of all pregnant mothers. However, some women may exhibit signs of an increased feeling of thirst, increased frequency of urination, feeling of fatigue, nausea and vomiting, infection in the bladder, infections by yeast and blurred vision.

Prevention

Prevention of Gestational Diabetes Mellitus is done by maintaining an ideal body weight and exercise regular exercise before the start of pregnancy (NIDDK, 2014). Gestational diabetes mellitus is managed with a diabetic diet, exercise and possibly injecting insulin (NIDDK, 2014). Blood sugar level is managed by most women through their diets and exercise (Donovan and McIntyre, 2010). For those who are affected, blood sugar testing is usually recommended four times a day (Donovan and McIntyre, 2010). Breastfeeding of the infant is recommended as soon as possible after birth (NIDDK, 2014).

Interventions for the management comprise of diet and physical activity which are aimed to reduce the rates of gestational diabetes mellitus by preventing excessive gestational weight gain. However, the effectiveness of these interventions depends upon the Body Mass Index (BMI) of the mother as well as with the region where the studies have been conducted (Bennett et al, 2018).

A 2015 review found that moderate physical exercise during pregnancy is effective for the prevention of gestational diabetes mellitus (Sanabria-Martínez et al, 2015). A 2014 review, however, did not find a significant effect of physical exercise for the prevention of gestational diabetes mellitus among pregnant women (Yin et al, 2014).

It has been further suggested that for women, who have had gestational diabetes mellitus in their previous pregnancy, support between pregnancies may lower their chances of having gestational diabetes mellitus again in their future pregnancies (Tieu et al, 2017). This support might include diet and physical exercise, education and lifestyle choices (Tieu et al, 2017). However, there is not much research evidence to show whether interventions between pregnancies lower the number of women who develop gestational diabetes mellitus again (Tieu et al, 2017).

Theoretically, smoking cessation may decrease the risk of gestational diabetes mellitus among pregnant women who smoke.

Treatment

Treatment of Gestational Diabetes Mellitus with diet and insulin reduces the health problems of both the mother and the child (Alwan et al, 2009). Treatment of Gestational Diabetes Mellitus is also accompanied by more inductions of labour (Alwan et al, 2009). A repeat Oral Glucose Tolerance Test (OGTT) should be undertaken at 6 weeks after delivery for confirming that diabetes mellitus has subsided. Thereafter, regular screening for type 2 diabetes mellitus is recommended (Ross, 2006).

Interventions for lifestyle changes include physical exercise, dietary counseling, behavior modification interventions, relaxation techniques, self-monitoring of glucose and/or a combination of these interventions (Brown et al, 2017). Research findings have revealed that when compared to women who had no intervention, pregnant women with gestational diabetes mellitus receiving lifestyle modification interventions had less postpartum depression and were more likely to achieve their targets of weight loss after giving birth (Brown et al, 2017). Their babies were also less likely to be large for their gestational age and had less percentage of fat when they were born (Brown et al, 2017).

If a diabetic diet or G.I. Diet, exercise and oral medication are inadequate to control glucose levels of pregnant women, insulin therapy may become necessary. Women who use insulin, with a history of stillbirth or with hypertension, are managed like women with overt diabetes (Precis, 1994).

Complications

Gestational Diabetes Mellitus (GDM) poses a high risk both to the mother as well as to the child. This risk is largely related to the uncontrolled blood glucose levels and its consequences to both mother and the child. The risk increases with higher blood glucose levels (Metzger et al, 2008).

Seventy percent of women with Gestational Diabetes Mellitus will develop Diabetes Mellitus at some point in their life and 40 to 50 percent of these women will develop Diabetes Mellitus within 10 years. Poorly controlled

Gestational Diabetes Mellitus places the foetus at a risk for adult onset of metabolic diseases (obesity, diabetes, hypertension, cardio-vascular diseases) (Denney and Quinn, 2018).

Treatment resulting in better control of these blood glucose levels can reduce some of the risks of Gestational Diabetes Mellitus considerably (Langer et al, 1994).

Infants

The two main risks which Gestational Diabetes Mellitus creates for the baby are the abnormalities in the growth pattern as well as chemical imbalances post birth, which require an immediate admission of the newborn to a Neonatal Intensive Care Unit (NICU). Mothers with Gestational Diabetes Mellitus give birth to infants who are at a risk of both bigger for their gestational age i.e. macrosomic (Metzger et al, 2008) in an unmanaged Gestational Diabetes Mellitus and small for their gestational age and intrauterine growth retardation (Setji et al, 2005) in the managed Gestational Diabetes Mellitus.

Further, Macrosomia leads to an increased risk of instrumental deliveries e.g. forceps, ventouse and caesarean section or problems in vaginal delivery such as shoulder dystocia. Macrosomia affects almost 12 percent of normal women as compared to 20 percent of women with Gestational Diabetes Mellitus (Kelly et al, 2005).

However, there is not very strong research evidence for each of these complications of infants. For example, in a study on Hyperglycemia and Adverse Pregnancy Outcome (HAPO), an increased risk for babies to be large but not small for gestational age was observed in women with uncontrolled Gestational Diabetes Mellitus (Metzger et al, 2008).

Research into complications for Gestational Diabetes Mellitus is difficult because of the many other confounding factors such as obesity and so on. Moreover, labeling a pregnant woman as having Gestational Diabetes Mellitus may in itself increase the risk of having an unnecessary caesarean section for the delivery (Naylor et al, 1997; Jovanovic-Peterson et al, 1997).

Neonates born to mothers with consistently high levels of blood sugar are also reported to be at a higher risk of low blood glucose i.e. hypoglycemia, jaundice, high red blood cell mass i.e. polycythemia and low level of calcium in blood i.e. hypocalcemia and low level of magnesium in blood i.e. hypomagnesemia (Jones, 2001). Besides, Gestational Diabetes Mellitus among pregnant women, if untreated, also interferes with the process of maturation of babies, causing dysmature babies who are more likely to be prone to incomplete lung maturation and impaired surfactant synthesis, thus leading to respiratory distress syndrome (Jones, 2001).

Gestational Diabetes Mellitus is not clearly shown as an independent risk factor for congenital defects, unlike pre-gestational diabetes mellitus. These defects usually emanate sometime during the first trimester i.e. before the 13th weeks of pregnancy whereas Gestational Diabetes Mellitus develops gradually. It is least pronounced during the first and early second trimester. It has been reported in studies that women with Gestational Diabetes Mellitus give birth to babies who are at an increased risk for congenital malformations (Allen and Armson, 2007; Martínez-Frías et al, 2005; Savona-Ventura and Gatt, 2004).

It was reported in a large case-control study that Gestational Diabetes Mellitus was associated with a limited group of birth defects. This association was usually limited to women with a high Body Mass Index ($BMI \geq 25\ kg/m^2$) (Correa et al, 2008). It is not easy to ensure that this is not partially as a result of inclusion of women with pre-existent type 2 diabetes mellitus those remained undiagnosed before pregnancy.

Due of various conflicting studies, it is not clear to conclude if pregnant women with Gestational Diabetes Mellitus are at an increased risk of preeclampsia (Leguizamón et al, 2006). In the Hyperglycemia and Adverse Pregnancy Outcome (HAPO) study, the risk of preeclampsia was between 13 percent and 37 percent higher although not all possible confounding factors were corrected (Metzger et al, 2008).

Ectopic Pregnancy

In the developed countries, the rate of ectopic pregnancy is about 1 to 2 percent of live births. It may be as high as 4 percent among those who make use of Assisted Reproductive Technology (ART) (Kirk et al, 2014). It is the commonest cause of mortality among women in first trimester of pregnancy at approximately 10 percent of the total deaths (Cecchino et al, 2014). In the developed world, the outcomes have improved while in the developing world, they often remain poor (Nama and Manyonda, 2009). The mortality risk is 0.1 to 0.3 percent in the developed world while it is between one to three percent in the developing world (Mignini, 2007).

Ectopic pregnancy is a pregnancy complication whereby an embryo attaches itself outside the uterus (Kirk et al, 2014). It's not always clear what causes an ectopic pregnancy. The symptoms linked to an ectopic pregnancy, in some cases, are inflammation and scarring of fallopian tubes from an earlier medical condition, infection or surgery, hormonal factors, genetic abnormalities, birth defects and medical conditions affecting the shape and condition of fallopian tubes and the organs of reproduction (Selner, 2018).

Classically, the signs and symptoms of ectopic pregnancy are abdominal pain and the vaginal bleeding (Crochet et al, 2013). Less than 50 percent of affected pregnant women reveal both symptoms (Crochet et al, 2013). The pain is usually described as sharp, dull or crampy (Crochet et al, 2013). If bleeding into the abdomen occurs, pain may also spread to the shoulders (Crochet et al, 2013). Severe bleeding may lead to a fast heart rate, fainting or shock (Kirk et al, 2014; Crochet et al, 2013). The foetus is unable to survive in rarer exceptions (Zhang et al, 2008).

The known description of ectopic pregnancy was first given in the 11th century by Al-Zahrawi (Nama, and Manyonda, 2009). The word "ectopic" means "out of place" (Cornog, 1998). It had been found that between 93 percent to 97 percent of ectopic pregnancies are located in a fallopian tube (Crochet et al, 2013). Of these, in turn, 13 percent are located in the isthmus, 75 percent in the ampulla and 12 percent in the fimbriae (Kirk et al, 2014). Ectopic pregnancy is accountable for almost 6 percent of maternal mortality in first trimester of pregnancy, making it the leading cause of maternal mortality in this stage of pregnancy (Crochet et al, 2013).

Again, women who were examined for ultrasound assessment with a positive pregnancy test reported that between 5 to 42 percent of them had a Pregnancy of Unknown Location (PUL), thereby indicating that there was a positive pregnancy test but no pregnancy was visualized at trans-vaginal ultrasonography (Kirk et al, 2014). It was also found that between 6 to 20 percent of Pregnancy of Unknown Location (PUL) were subsequently diagnosed with actual ectopic pregnancy (Kirk et al, 2014).

Risk Factors

Risk factors associated with ectopic pregnancy are pelvic inflammatory disease, often due to Chlamydia infection, tobacco smoking, prior tubal surgery, a history of infertility and the use of Assisted Reproductive Technology (ART) (Cecchino et al, 2014). Those women with a previous history of ectopic pregnancy are at higher risk of another one (Cecchino et al, 2014).

Most ectopic pregnancies (90%) occur in the fallopian tube, also called tubal pregnancies (Cecchino et al, 2014). Implantation may also occur in the cervix, ovaries or within the abdomen (Crochet et al, 2013). Other causes of similar symptoms may include miscarriage, ovarian torsion and acute appendicitis etc. (Crochet et al, 2013).

Signs and Symptoms

It has been reported that up to 10 percent of women with ectopic pregnancy reveal no symptoms and one third reveal any medical signs (Kirk et al, 2014). The symptoms of ectopic pregnancy have very low specificity in many cases and quite resemble to those of genito-urinary and gastro-intestinal disorders such as appendicitis, salpingitis and rupture of a corpus luteum cyst, miscarriage, ovarian torsion or urinary tract infection (Kirk et al, 2014). However, the clinical manifestation of ectopic pregnancy symptoms usually occurs at a mean period of 7.2 weeks following the normal last menstrual period, with a range of four to eight weeks. Later manifestations of ectopic pregnancy symptoms are quite common in communities or regions which are devoid of modern diagnostic technology.

Other signs and symptoms of ectopic pregnancy are an increased hCG, bleeding from vaginal (in varying amounts), sudden pain in lower abdominal (Kirk et al, 2014), pelvic pain, a tender cervix, an adnexal mass or adnexal tenderness (Crochet et al, 2013).

In the absence of an ultrasound or hCG assessment, heavy vaginal bleeding during pregnancy may result in a misdiagnosis of miscarriage (Kirk et al, 2014). Nausea, vomiting and diarrhoea are rare symptoms of ectopic pregnancy (Kirk et al, 2014). A rupture of the ectopic pregnancy can result in symptoms such as abdominal distension, tenderness, peritonism and hypovolemic shock for the women (Kirk et al, 2014).

A woman with ectopic pregnancy may be excessively mobile with upright posture to decrease intra-pelvic blood flow, leading to abdominal cavity swelling and further pain (Skipworth, 2011).

Diagnosis

Detection of ectopic pregnancy is typically through the blood tests for human chorionic gonadotropin (hCG) and assessment through an ultrasound (Crochet et al, 2013). This may require testing on more than one occasion (Crochet et al, 2013). Ultrasound works best when performed from within the vagina (Crochet et al, 2013).

Prevention

Prevention of ectopic pregnancy can be done by decreasing the risk factors such as Chlamydia infections through regular screening and treatment (Nama and Manyonda, 2009). While some of the ectopic pregnancies resolve without treatment, this approach has not been well studied as of the year 2014 (Cecchino et al, 2014).

The use of medication i.e. methotrexate works well and a surgery in other cases (Cecchino et al, 2014). Specifically, it works well if beta-HCG (beta-Human Chorionic Gonadotropin) hormone level is low and the ectopic size is small (Cecchino et al, 2014). Surgery is still recommended if the tube has ruptured, there is a fetal heartbeat or the mother's vital signs are not stable (Cecchino et al, 2014). Surgery may be laparoscopic or through a larger incision, called laparotomy (Kirk et al, 2014). However, the outcomes of ectopic pregnancy are generally good with appropriate and timely treatment (Cecchino et al, 2014).

Complication

The commonest complication of ectopic pregnancy may lead to hypovolemic shock for the mother due to rupture with internal bleeding. In the first trimester of the pregnancy, death due to rupture is the leading cause of maternal mortality (Rastogi, 2017; Pediatric Clinical Advisor, 2007; Tenore, 2000).

Miscarriage

Miscarriage is the most common complication of early pregnancy (National Coordinating Centre for Women's and Children's Health, 2012). Among women knowing they are pregnant, the rate of miscarriage is nearly 10 to 20 percent while rate among all fertilizations is around 30 to 50 percent (Lippincott Williams and Wilkins, 2012; NICHD, 2013). About 5 percent of women have two miscarriages in succession (Garrido-Gimenez and Alijotas-Reig, 2015). It has been recommended not to use the term "abortion" while discussing with those undergone a miscarriage in an effort to decrease distress among women (Greaves et al, 2005).

Miscarriage, also known as spontaneous abortion or loss of pregnancy, is the natural death of an embryo or foetus before it is able to survive independently (Lippincott Williams and Wilkins, 2012; NICHD, 2013). Some use the cut-off period of 20 weeks of gestation, following which foetal death is called a stillbirth (National Institute of child Health and Human Development (NICHD, 2013). The commonest symptom of a miscarriage is bleeding from vagina with or without pain (Lippincott Williams and Wilkins, 2012). Tissues and a clot-like material may leave the uterus and pass through and out of the vagina (NICHD, 2013). Sadness, anxiety and guilt usually occur afterwards (Robinson, 2014; NICHD, 2013). When a woman undergoes repeated miscarriages, infertility is likely to occur (womenshealth, 2017).

First Trimester

Most clinically apparent miscarriages (two-thirds to three-quarters reported in various studies) occur during first trimester (Lippincott Williams and Wilkins, 2012; Rosenthal, 1999; (Cunningham et al, 2013). About 30 to 40 percent of all fertilized eggs undergo miscarriage, often before the pregnancy is known (Lippincott Williams and Wilkins, 2012). The embryo typically dies before it is expelled; bleeding into the decidua basalis and tissue necrosis causes uterine contractions to expel the embryo (Cunningham et al, 2013).

Early miscarriages during first trimester may be due to abnormality in the development of the placenta or other embryonic tissues. In some cases, other tissues do form but an embryo does not form. This is called a "blighted ovum" (American Pregnancy Association, 2012; Mayo Clinic, 2017).

Implantation of zygote successfully into the uterus is likely to occur from 8 to 10 days after the conception. If the zygote has not been implanted by day 10 after fertilization, implantation becomes increasingly unlikely in subsequent days of pregnancy (Wilcox et al, 1999).

Moreover, there are chromosomal abnormalities present in more than half of the embryos which are miscarried in the first 13 weeks of gestation. Half of embryonic miscarriages (25 percent of total miscarriages) have an aneuploidy (abnormal number of chromosomes) (Kajii et al, 1980). Common chromosomal abnormalities present in miscarriages are an autosomal trisomy (22 to 32 percent), monosomy X (5 to 20 percent), triploidy (6 to 8 percent), tetraploidy (2 to 4 percent) or other structural chromosomal abnormalities (2 percent) (Cunningham et al, 2013).

Genetic problems are, however, more likely to occur with older parents and this may account for the higher rates of miscarriages observed in older women (MUSC Children's Hospital, 2006).

Second and Third Trimesters

During the second trimester, various maternal factors such as uterine malformation, growths in the uterus (fibroids) or cervical problems may lead to losses (NHS, 2017). These conditions may also lead to preterm birth (Rosenthal, 1999). Second-trimester miscarriages are less likely to be caused due to genetic abnormality unlike first-trimester miscarriages; chromosomal aberrations are found in almost one-third of all cases (Cunningham et al, 2013). Infection during the third trimester can also cause a miscarriage (NHS, 2017).

Etiology

A 2012 review found the risk of miscarriage between 5th and 20th weeks of gestation rises from 11 percent to 22 percent (Ammon et al, 2012). The risk of miscarriage per week was around 2 percent up to the 13th week of pregnancy, it dropped to 1 percent in 14th week and reduced slowly from 14th to 20th week of gestation (Ammon et al, 2012).

The precise rate of miscarriages is unknown because a number of miscarriages take place before pregnancies are established and before the women are aware of the fact that they are pregnant (Ammon et al, 2012). Additionally, women experiencing bleeding in early pregnancy seek medical help more often than those not experiencing bleeding (Ammon et al, 2012). Although attempts have been made in some studies to account for this by recruiting women planning their pregnancies and testing for very early pregnancy but those were still not the representative sample of the wider population (Ammon et al, 2012).

Moreover, the prevalence of miscarriage increases with the increasing age of both parents (Ammon et al, 2012; Kleinhaus et al, 2006; Slama et al, 2005). In a register-based Danish study where the rate of prevalence of miscarriage was 11 percent, the prevalence rate rose from 9 to 84 percent from 22 years to 48 years of age (Nybo et al, 2000). Later, another study undertaken in 2013 found that when either parent was above 40 years, the rate of known miscarriages was doubled (Cunningham et al, 2013).

Risk Factors

There are many reasons why miscarriage may occur, not all of which can be identified. Risk factors are those things that increase the probability of a miscarriage but do not necessarily cause a miscarriage. Up to 70 conditions (Lippincott Williams and Wilkins, 2012; Vaiman, 2015; Ali et al, 2015; Tersigni et al, 2014), infections (NHS, 2017; American College of Obstetricians and Gynecologists, 2014; Lis et al, 2015), medical procedures (Tabor and Alfirevic, 2010; Agarwal and Alfirevic, 2012; Alfirevic et al, 2017), lifestyle factors (NICHD, 2013; Oliver and Overton, 2014; Ness et al, 1999; NHS, 2017; Venners et al, 2004) occupational exposures (NICHD, 2013), chemical exposure and shift work are associated with an increased risk for miscarriage (Chavarro et al, 2016). Some of the risk factors are genetic, endocrine, uterine or hormonal abnormalities, reproductive tract infections and tissue rejection caused by an auto-immune disorder (Acién and Acién, 2016).

Other significant risk factors for miscarriages include older parents, previous history of miscarriages, an exposure to tobacco or smoking, obesity, diabetes mellitus, thyroid problems and drug or alcohol use (NICHD, 2013; Oliver and Overton, 2014).

The age of the pregnant woman is also a significant risk factor. The rates of miscarriage increase steadily with age, with more substantial increase after the age of 35 years (Bray et al, 2006). In those under 35 years of age, the risk is about 10 percent while it is about 45 percent in those over the age of 40 years (Lippincott Williams and Wilkins, 2012). Risk begins to increase around the age of 30 years (NICHD, 2013). Paternal age is associated with an increased risk.

About 80 percent of miscarriages take place in the first 12 weeks of gestation i.e. the first trimester (Lippincott Williams and Wilkins, 2012). The underlying cause of about half of the miscarriages involves chromosomal abnormalities (Vaiman, 2015; Lippincott Williams and Wilkins, 2012). Other conditions producing similar symptoms are an ectopic pregnancy and an implantation bleeding (Lippincott Williams and Wilkins, 2012).

Signs

Signs of a miscarriage are vaginal spotting, abdominal pain, cramping and fluid, blood clots and tissues passing from the vagina (NICHD, 2017; Li et al, 2012). Bleeding may represent a symptom of miscarriage. In early pregnancy, though, many women also have bleeding but they don't miscarry. Bleeding during pregnancy could be considered as a threatened miscarriage. Of those women seeking treatment for bleeding during pregnancy, approximately half miscarry (Everett, 1997).

Diagnosis

Diagnosis of a miscarriage may involve examination to check if the cervix is open or closed, testing the levels of human chorionic gonadotropin (hCG) in blood and an ultrasound (NICHD, 2013).

Prevention

Prevention of miscarriage is occasionally possible if there is good prenatal care (NICHD, 2013). The risk of miscarriage may be decreased by avoiding drugs, alcohol, infectious diseases and radiation (NICHD, 2013). There is, however, no evidence to prove that progesterone reduces the risk of miscarriage if given in the first trimester. The luteal phase progesterone deficiency may or may not be a contributing factor of miscarriage (Wahabi et al, 2011; Bukulmez and Arici, 2004).

Treatment

No specific treatment is often required during the first 7 to 14 days (Oliver and Overton, 2014; NICHD, 2013). Most miscarriages will complete without additional interventions (Oliver and Overton, 2014). Occasionally, the medication or a procedure involving vacuum aspiration is used to remove the remaining tissues (www.nichd.nih.gov, 2013; Tunçalp et al, 2010). Women whose blood type is rhesus negative (Rh negative) may require Rho (D) immune globulin (Oliver and Overton, 2014). Medication for pain may be beneficial (NICHD, 2013). Emotional support may help with the recovering the loss (NICHD, 2013).

CONCLUSION

Whether the complications of pregnancy are common or rare, there are always ways to manage the problems that come up during pregnancy. Although many complications are mild and are not progressive but one should always consult the gynecologist if one has any concerns during pregnancy. Most pregnancy complications are manageable with early identification and prompt treatment. Getting early and regular antenatal chekup can help decrease the risk for complications by enabling the health care providers to identify, diagnose, treat or manage the complications before they become serious and are threat to pregnancy. Even with complications, early detection and antenatal care can reduce any further risk to the health of mother and the newborn and hence decrease the maternal and neonatal mortality and morbidity rates.

REFERENCES

Acién, P., & Acién, M. (2016). The presentation and management of complex female genital malformations. *Human Reproduction Update, 22*(1), 48–69. doi:10.1093/humupd/dmv048

ACOG (American College of Obstetrics and Gynecology). (2016). *Multiple Pregnancy - ACOG.* www.acog.org

Agarwal, K., & Alfirevic, Z. (2012). Pregnancy loss after chorionic villus sampling and genetic amniocentesis in twin pregnancies: A systematic review. *Ultrasound in Obstetrics & Gynecology, 40*(2), 128–134. doi:10.1002/uog.10152 PMID:22125091

Ahmed, K. T., Almashhrawi, A. A., Rahman, R. N., Hammoud, G. M., & Ibdah, J. A. (2013). Liver diseases in pregnancy: Diseases unique to pregnancy. *World Journal of Gastroenterology, 19*(43), 7639–7646. doi:10.3748/wjg.v19.i43.7639 PMID:24282353

Alexander, G. R., Kogan, M., Martin, J., & Papiernik, E. (1998). What are the fetal growth patterns of singletons, twins, and triplets in the United States? *Clinical Obstetrics and Gynecology, 41*(1), 114–125. doi:10.1097/00003081-199803000-00017 PMID:9504230

Alfirevic, Z., Navaratnam, K. & Mujezinovic, F. (2017). *Cochrane database of systematic reviews.* John Wiley & Sons, Ltd. doi:10.1002/14651858.cd003252.pub2

Ali, O., Hakimi, I., Chanana, A., Habib, M., Abdellah, B., Guelzim, K., Kouach, J., Rahali, D., Moussaoui, & Dehayeni, M. (2015). Term pegnancy on septate uterus: report of a case and review of the literature. *The Pan African Medical Journal, 22*, 219. doi:10.11604/pamj.2015.22.219.7790

Allen, V. M., Armson, B. A., Wilson, R. D., Allen, V. M., Blight, C., Gagnon, A., Johnson, J.-A., Langlois, S., Summers, A., Wyatt, P., Farine, D., Armson, B. A., Crane, J., Delisle, M.-F., Keenan-Lindsay, L., Morin, V., Schneider, C. E., & Van Aerde, J. (2007). Teratogenicity associated with pre-existing and gestational diabetes. *Journal of Obstetrics and Gynaecology Canada, 29*(11), 927–934. doi:10.1016/S1701-2163(16)32653-6 PMID:17977497

Alwan, N., Tuffnell, D. J., & West, J. (2009). Treatments for gestational diabetes. *Cochrane Database of Systematic Reviews*, (3), CD003395. doi:10.1002/14651858.CD003395.pub2 PMID:19588341

American College of Obstetricians and Gynecologists. (2014). ACOG Practice Bulletin No.142: Cerclage for the management of cervical insufficiency. *Obstetrics and Gynecology, 123*(2 Pt 1), 372–379. doi:10.1097/01.AOG.0000443276.68274.cc PMID:24451674

American Diabetes Association. (2004). Gestational diabetes mellitus. *Diabetes Care, 27*(1), S88–S90. doi:10.2337/diacare.27.2007.s88 PMID:14693936

American Pregnancy Association. (2012). *Blighted Ovum: Symptoms, Causes and Prevention*. APA.

Ammon, A. L., Galindo, C., & Li, D. K. (2012). A systematic review to calculate background miscarriage rates using life table analysis. *Birth Defects Research. Part A, Clinical and Molecular Teratology, 94*(6), 417–423. doi:10.1002/bdra.23014 PMID:22511535

Beemsterboer, S. N., Homburg, R., Gorter, N. A., Schats, R., Hompes, P. G., & Lambalk, C. B. (2006). The paradox of declining fertility but increasing twinning rates with advancing maternal age. *Human Reproduction (Oxford, England), 21*(6), 1531–1532. doi:10.1093/humrep/del009 PMID:16497698

Bennett, C. J., Walker, R. E., Blumfield, M. L., Gwini, S. M., Ma, J., Wang, F., Wan, Y., Dickinson, H., & Truby, H. (2018). Interventions designed to reduce excessive gestational weight gain can reduce the incidence of gestational diabetes mellitus: A systematic review and meta-analysis of randomised controlled trials. *Diabetes Research and Clinical Practice (Review), 141*, 69–79. doi:10.1016/j.diabres.2018.04.010 PMID:29698713

Bjørge, T., Tretli, S., & Engeland, A. (2004). Relation of height and body mass index to renal cell carcinoma in two million Norwegian men and women. *American Journal of Epidemiology*, *160*(12), 1168–1176. doi:10.1093/aje/kwh345 PMID:15583369

Borders, N. (2006). After the afterbirth: A critical review of postpartum health relative to method of delivery. *Journal of Midwifery & Women's Health*, *51*(4), 242–248. doi:10.1016/j.jmwh.2005.10.014 PMID:16814217

Bourne, T. H. & Condous, G. (Eds.). (2006). Handbook of early pregnancy care: Information Healthcare. Academic Press.

Bray, I., Gunnell, D., & Davey Smith, G. (2006). Advanced paternal age: How old is too old? *Journal of Epidemiology and Community Health*, *60*(10), 851–853. doi:10.1136/jech.2005.045179 PMID:16973530

Brown, J., Alwan, N. A., West, J., Brown, S., McKinlay, C. J., Farrar, D., & Crowther, C. A. (2017). Lifestyle interventions for the treatment of women with gestational diabetes. *Cochrane Database of Systematic Reviews*, *5*. doi:10.1002/14651858.CD011970.pub2 PMID:28472859

Bukulmez, O. & Arici, A. (2004). Luteal phase defect: Myth or reality? *Obstetrics and Gynecology Clinics of North America, 31*(4), 727–44. doi:10.1016/j.ogc.2004.08.007

Carlson, K. J., Eisenstat, S. J., & Ziporyn, T. (2004). The New Harvard Guide to Women's Health. Harvard University Press.

Cecchino, G. N., Araujo Júnior, E., & Elito Júnior, J. (2014). Methotrexate for ectopic pregnancy: When and how. *Archives of Gynecology and Obstetrics*, *290*(3), 417–423. doi:10.100700404-014-3266-9 PMID:24791968

Centers for Disease Control and Prevention. (2007). *Preventing smoking and exposure to secondhand smoke before, during and after pregnancy*. Academic Press.

Centers for Disease Control and Prevention (2009). *Tobacco Use and Pregnancy: Home*. Author.

Centre for Disease Control (2015). *Severe Maternal Morbidity in the United States*. CDC.

Chavarro, J. E., Rich-Edwards, J. W., Gaskins, A. J., Farland, L. V., Terry, K. L., Zhang, C., & Missmer, S. A. (2016). Contributions of the nurses' health studies to reproductive health research. *American Journal of Public Health, 106*(9), 1669–1676. doi:10.2105/AJPH.2016.303350

Christodoulou-Smith, J., Gold, J. I., Romero, R., Goodwin, T. M., Macgibbon, K. W., Mullin, P. M., & Fejzo, M. S. (2011). Posttraumatic stress symptoms following pregnancy complicated by hyperemesis gravidarum. *The Journal of Maternal-Fetal & Neonatal Medicine*, *24*(11), 1307–1311. doi:10.3109/14767058.2011.582904 PMID:21635201

Chu, S. Y., Callaghan, W. M., Kim, S. Y., Schmid, C. H., Lau, J., England, L. J., & Dietz, P. M. (2007). Maternal obesity and risk of gestational diabetes mellitus. *Diabetes Care*, *30*(8), 2070–2076. doi:10.2337/dc06-2559a PMID:17416786

Cornog, M. W. (1998). Merriam-Webster's vocabulary Builder. Springfield, MA: Merriam-Webster.

Correa, A., Gilboa, S. M., Besser, L. M., Botto, L. D., Moore, C. A., Hobbs, C. A., Cleves, M. A., Riehle-Colarusso, T. J., Waller, D. K., & Reece, E. A. (2008). Diabetes mellitus and birth defects. *American Journal of Obstetrics and Gynecology*, *199*(3), 237.e1–237.e9. doi:10.1016/j.ajog.2008.06.028 PMID:18674752

Crochet, J. R., Bastian, L. A., & Chireau, M. V. (2013). Does this woman have an ectopic pregnancy?: The rational clinical examination systematic review. *Journal of the American Medical Association*, *309*(16), 1722–1729. doi:10.1001/jama.2013.3914 PMID:23613077

Cunningham, F., Leveno, K. J., Bloom, S. L., Spong, C. Y., Dashe, J. S., Hoffman, B. L., Casey, B. M., & Sheffield, J. S. (2013). *Abortion. Williams Obstetrics*. McGraw-Hill.

DeLegge, M. H. (2007). Handbook of home nutrition support. Sudbury, MA: Jones and Bartlett.

Della Grotta, S., LaGasse, L. L., Arria, A. M., Derauf, C., Grant, P., Smith, L. M., Shah, R., Huestis, M., Liu, J., & Lester, B. M. (2010). Patterns of methamphetamine use during pregnancy: Results from the Infant Development, Environment, and Lifestyle (IDEAL) Study. *Maternal and Child Health Journal*, *14*(4), 519–527. doi:10.100710995-009-0491-0 PMID:19565330

Denney, J. M., & Quinn, K. H. (2018). Gestational Diabetes. *Obstretics and Gynecology Clinics, 45*(2), 299–314. PMID:29747732

Dodds, L., Fell, D. B., Joseph, K. S., Allen, V. M., & Butler, B. (2006). Outcomes of pregnancies complicated by hyperemesis gravidarum. *Obstetrics and Gynecology, 107*(2 Pt 1), 285–292. doi:10.1097/01.AOG.0000195060.22832.cd PMID:16449113

Donovan, P. J., & McIntyre, H. D. (2010). Drugs for gestational diabetes. *Australian Prescriber, 33*(5), 141–144. doi:10.18773/austprescr.2010.066

Eisenberg, L., & Brown, S. H. (1995). The best intentions: unintended pregnancy and the well-being of children and families. Washington, DC: National Academy Press.

Evans, A. T. (Ed.). (2007). Manual of obstetrics (7th ed.). Wolters Kluwer / Lippincott Williams & Wilkins.

Everett, C. (1997). Incidence and outcome of bleeding before the 20th week of pregnancy: Prospective study from general practice. *British Medical Journal, 315*(7099), 32–4. doi:10.1136/bmj.315.7099.32

Family Planning- Healthy People (2020). Archived from the original on 20010-12-28. Retrieved 2011-08-18.

Fejzo, M.S., Magtira, A., Schoenberg, F.P., Macgibbon, K. & Mullin, P.M. (2015). Neurodevelopmental delay in children exposed in utero to hyperemesis gravidarum. *European Journal of Obstetrics & Gynecology and Reproduction Biology, 189*, 79–84. doi:10.1016/j.ejogrb.2015.03.028

Ferri, F. F. (2012). Ferri's Clinical Advisor 2013 5 books in 1. Elsevier Mosby.

Gabbe, S. G. (2012). Obstetrics: Normal and problem pregnancies (6th ed.). Elsevier/Saunders.

Garrido-Gimenez, C., & Alijotas-Reig, J. (2015). Recurrent miscarriage: Causes, evaluation and management. *Postgraduate Medical Journal, 91*(1073), 151–162. doi:10.1136/postgradmedj-2014-132672 PMID:25681385

Gavin, A. R., Holzman, C., Siefert, K., & Tian, Y. (2009). Maternal depressive symptoms, depression, and psychiatric medication use in relation to risk of preterm delivery. *Women's Health Issues, 19*(5), 325–334. doi:10.1016/j.whi.2009.05.004 PMID:19733802

Glazener, C. M., Abdalla, M., Stroud, P., Naji, S., Templeton, A., & Russell, I. T. (1995). Postnatal maternal morbidity: Extent, causes, prevention and treatment. *British Journal of Obstetrics and Gynaecology*, *102*(4), 282–287. doi:10.1111/j.1471-0528.1995.tb09132.x PMID:7612509

Global Burden of Disease. (2016). Causes of Death Collaborators (September 2017). Global, regional, and national age-sex specific mortality for 264 causes of death, 1980-2016: A systematic analysis for the Global Burden of Disease Study 2016. *Lancet*, *390*(10100), 1151–1210. doi:10.1016/S0140-6736(17)32152-9

Glossary. (2017). www.womenshealth.gov

Goodwin, T.M. (2008). Hyperemesis gravidarum. *Obstetrics and Gynecology Clinics of North America, 35*(3), 401–17. doi:10.1016/j.ogc.2008.04.002

Greaves, I., Porter, K., Hodgetts, T. J., & Woollard, M. (2005). *Emergency Care: A Textbook for Paramedics*. London: Elsevier Health Sciences.

Hammond, K. R. (1998). Multifetal pregnancy reduction. *Journal of Obstetric, Gynecologic, and Neonatal Nursing*, *27*(3), 338–343. doi:10.1111/j.1552-6909.1998.tb02657.x PMID:9620827

How do health care providers diagnose pregnancy loss or miscarriage? (2013). www.nichd.nih.gov/

How do health care providers diagnose pregnancy loss or miscarriage? (2017). www.nichd.nih.gov

How many people are affected by or at risk for pregnancy loss or miscarriage? (2013). www.nichd.nih.gov

Is there a cure for pregnancy loss/miscarriage? (2015). www.nichd.nih.gov/

Jones, C. W. (2001). Gestational diabetes and its impact on the neonate. *Neonatal Network*, *20*(6), 17–23. doi:10.1891/0730-0832.20.6.17 PMID:12144115

Jovanovic-Peterson, L., Bevier, W., & Peterson, C. M. (1997). The Santa Barbara County Health Care Services program: birth weight change concomitant with screening for and treatment of glucose-intolerance of pregnancy: a potential cost-effective intervention? *American Journal of Perinatology*, *14*(4), 221–228. doi:10.1055-2007-994131 PMID:9259932

Jueckstock, J. K., Kaestner, R., & Mylonas, I. (2010). Managing hyperemesis gravidarum: A multimodal challenge. *BioMed Central Medicine*, *8*, 46. doi:10.1186/1741-7015-8-46 PMID:20633258

Kajii, T., Ferrier, A., Niikawa, N., Takahara, H., Ohama, K., & Avirachan, S. (1980). Anatomic and chromosomal anomalies in 639 spontaneous abortuses. *Human Genetics*, *55*(1), 87–98. doi:10.1007/BF00329132 PMID:7450760

Kelly, L., Evans, L., & Messenger, D. (2005). Controversies around gestational diabetes. Practical information for family doctors. *Canadian Family Physician Medecin de Famille Canadien*, *51*(5), 688–695. PMID:15934273

Khandwala, Y. S., Baker, V. L., Shaw, G. M., Stevenson, D. K., Lu, Y., & Eisenberg, M. L. (2018). Association of paternal age with perinatal outcomes between 2007 and 2016 in the United States: Population based cohort study. *British Medical Journal*, *363*, k4372. doi:10.1136/bmj.k4372 PMID:30381468

Kirk, E., Bottomley, C., & Bourne, T. (2014). Diagnosing ectopic pregnancy and current concepts in the management of pregnancy of unknown location. *Human Reproduction Update*, *20*(2), 250–261. doi:10.1093/humupd/dmt047 PMID:24101604

Kleinhaus, K., Perrin, M., Friedlander, Y., Paltiel, O., Malaspina, D., & Harlap, S. (2006). Paternal Age and Spontaneous Abortion. *Obstetrics and Gynecology*, *108*(2), 369–377. doi:10.1097/01.AOG.0000224606.26514.3a PMID:16880308

Kumar, G. (2011). Early Pregnancy Issues for the MRCOG and Beyond. Cambridge University Press. doi:10.1017/CBO9781139696975

Langer, O., Rodriguez, D. A., Xenakis, E. M., McFarland, M. B., Berkus, M. D., & Arrendondo, F. (1994). Intensified versus conventional management of gestational diabetes. *American Journal of Obstetrics and Gynecology*, *170*(4), 1036–1046. doi:10.1016/S0002-9378(94)70097-4 PMID:8166187

Le, J. (2011). *Scale-tipping triplets set world record*. Mississauga News.

Leguizamón, G. F., Zeff, N. P., & Fernández, A. (2006). Hypertension and the pregnancy complicated by diabetes. *Current Diabetes Reports*, *6*(4), 297–304. doi:10.100711892-006-0064-1 PMID:16879782

Levi, J., Kohn, D. & Johnson, K. (2011). *Healthy Women, Healthy Babies: How health reform can improve the health of women and babies in America*. Washington, DC: Trust for America's Health.

Li, L., Dou, L., Leung, P. C., & Wang, C. C. (2012). Chinese herbal medicines for threatened miscarriage. *Cochrane Database of Systematic Reviews*, (5), CD008510. doi:10.1002/14651858.cd008510.pub2 PMID:22592730

Lippincott, Williams & Wilkins. (2012). *The Johns Hopkins Manual of Gynecology and Obstetrics* (4th ed.). Author.

Lis, R., Rowhani-Rahbar, A., & Manhart, L. E. (2015). Mycoplasma genitalium infection and female reproductive tract disease: A meta-analysis. *Clinical Infectious Diseases, 61*(3), 418–26. doi:10.1093/cid/civ312

Ma, R. M., Lao, T. T., Ma, C. L., Liao, S. J., Lu, Y. F., Du, M. Y., Xiao, H., Zhang, L., Yang, M. H., & Xiao, X. (2007). Relationship between leg length and gestational diabetes mellitus in Chinese pregnant women. *Diabetes Care, 30*(11), 2960–2961. doi:10.2337/dc07-0763 PMID:17666468

Management of Hyperemesis Gravidarum. (2013). ▼Linaclotide for constipation-predominant IBS. *Drug and Therapeutics Bulletin, 51*(11), 129–9. doi:10.1136/dtb.2013.11.0218 PMID:24227771

Martínez-Frías, M. L., Frías, J. P., Bermejo, E., Rodríguez-Pinilla, E., Prieto, L., & Frías, J. L. (2005). Pre-gestational maternal body mass index predicts an increased risk of congenital malformations in infants of mothers with gestational diabetes. *Diabetic Medicine, 22*(6), 775–781. doi:10.1111/j.1464-5491.2005.01492.x PMID:15910631

Matthews, A., Haas, D. M., O'Mathúna, D. P., & Dowswell, T. (2015). Interventions for nausea and vomiting in early pregnancy. *The Cochrane Database of Systematic Reviews*, (9). doi:10.1002/14651858.CD007575.pub4

Matthews, D. C., & Syed, A. A. (2011). The role of TSH receptor antibodies in the management of Graves' disease. *European Journal of Internal Medicine, 22*(3), 213–216. doi:10.1016/j.ejim.2011.02.006 PMID:21570635

Mayo Clinic (2017). *Blighted ovum: What causes it?* Author.

Merck Sharp & Dohme (2013). Risk factors present before pregnancy. In *Merck Manual Home Health Handbook*. Author.

Metzger, B.E. & Coustan, D.R. (1998). Summary and recommendations of the Fourth International Workshop-Conference on Gestational Diabetes Mellitus. *The Organizing Committee. Diabetes Care, 21*(2), B161–7.

Metzger, B. E., Lowe, L. P., Dyer, A. R., Trimble, E. R., Chaovarindr, U., Coustan, D. R., Hadden, D. R., McCance, D. R., Hod, M., McIntyre, H. D., Oats, J. J., Persson, B., Rogers, M. S., & Sacks, D. A. (2008). Hyperglycemia and adverse pregnancy outcomes. *The New England Journal of Medicine*, *358*(19), 1991–2002. doi:10.1056/NEJMoa0707943 PMID:18463375

Mignini, L. (2007). *Interventions for tubal ectopic pregnancy*. WHO International.

MUSC Children's Hospital. (2006). *Pregnancy Over Age 30*. Author.

Nama, V., & Manyonda, I. (2009). Tubal ectopic pregnancy: Diagnosis and management. *Archives of Gynecology and Obstetrics*, *279*(4), 443–453. doi:10.100700404-008-0731-3 PMID:18665380

National Coordinating Centre for Women's and Children's Health (UK). (2012). *Ectopic Pregnancy and Miscarriage: Diagnosis and Initial Management in Early Pregnancy of Ectopic Pregnancy and Miscarriage*. NICE Clinical Guidelines, No. 154. Royal College of Obstetricians and Gynaecologists.

Naylor, C. D., Sermer, M., Chen, E., & Farine, D. (1997). Selective screening for gestational diabetes mellitus. Toronto Trihospital Gestational Diabetes Project Investigators. *The New England Journal of Medicine*, *337*(22), 1591–1596. doi:10.1056/NEJM199711273372204 PMID:9371855

Neilson, J. P., West, H. M., & Dowswell, T. (2014). Betamimetics for inhibiting preterm labour. *Cochrane Database of Systematic Reviews*, *2*(2). doi:10.1002/14651858.CD004352.pub3 PMID:24500892

Ness, R. B., Grisso, J. A., Hirschinger, N., Markovic, N., Shaw, L. M., Day, N. L., & Kline, J. (1999). Cocaine and Tobacco Use and the Risk of Spontaneous Abortion. *The New England Journal of Medicine*, *340*(5), 333–339. doi:10.1056/NEJM199902043400501 PMID:9929522

NHS. (2017). *Choices, Miscarriage - Causes - NHS Choices*. www.nhs.uk

NICE (National Institute for Clinical Excellence). (2011). *Glossary: Multiple pregnancy: antenatal care for twin and triplet pregnancies*. NICE.

NICHD (National Institute of Child Health and Human Development). (2014). *Stillbirth: Overview*. NICHD.

NIDDK (National Institute of Diabetes and Digestive and Kidney Diseases). (2014). *Gestational Diabetes*. NIDDK.

Niebyl, J. R. (2010). Nausea and Vomiting in Pregnancy. *The New England Journal of Medicine*, *363*(16), 1544–1550. doi:10.1056/NEJMcp1003896 PMID:20942670

Norris, S. A., Osmond, C., Gigante, D., Kuzawa, C. W., Ramakrishnan, L., Lee, N. R., Ramirez-Zea, M., Richter, L. M., Stein, A. D., Tandon, N., & Fall, C. H. D. (2012). Size at birth, weight gain in infancy and childhood, and adult diabetes risk in five low- or middle-income country birth cohorts. *Diabetes Care*, *35*(1), 72–79. doi:10.2337/dc11-0456 PMID:22100968

North Dakota Department of Health (2011). *New Mother Fact Sheet: Methamphetamine Use During Pregnancy*. Author.

Nybo Andersen, A.M., Wohlfahrt, J., Christens, P., Olsen, J. & Melbye, M. (2000). Maternal age and fetal loss: Population based register linkage study. *BMJ, 320*(7251), 1708–12. doi:10.1136/bmj.320.7251.1708

Office on Women's Health (2010). *Pregnancy.* Author.

Oliver, A. & Overton, C. (2014). Diagnosis and management of miscarriage. *The Practitioner, 258*(1771), 25–8.

Pediatric Clinical Advisor. (2007). Instant Diagnosis and Treatment (2nd ed.). Mosby Elsevier.

Precis, V. (1994). An Update on Obstetrics and Gynecology. American College of Obstetrics and Gynecology.

Rafael, T. J., Berghella, V., & Alfirevic, Z. (2014). Cervical stitch (cerclage) for preventing preterm birth in multiple pregnancy. *Cochrane Database of Systematic Reviews*, *9*(9), CD009166. doi:10.1002/14651858.CD009166.pub2 PMID:25208049

Rastogi, A. (2017). *Ectopic pregnancy*. Academic Press.

Robinson, G. E. (2014). Pregnancy loss. *Best Practice & Research. Clinical Obstetrics & Gynaecology*, *28*(1), 169–178. doi:10.1016/j.bpobgyn.2013.08.012 PMID:24047642

Rosenthal, M. S. (1999). The Second Trimester. In *The Gynecological Sourcebook*. WebMD.

Ross, G. (2006). Gestational diabetes. *Australian Family Physician*, *35*(6), 392–396. PMID:16751853

Ross, J., John, S., & Amy, W. (1999). *Profiles for family planning and reproductive health programs in 116 countries*. The Futures Group International.

Sanabria-Martínez, G., García-Hermoso, A., Poyatos-León, R., Álvarez-Bueno, C., Sánchez-López, M., & Martínez-Vizcaíno, V. (2015). Effectiveness of physical activity interventions on preventing gestational diabetes mellitus and excessive maternal weight gain: A meta-analysis. *British Journal of Obstetrics and Gynaecology*, *122*(9), 1167–1174. doi:10.1111/1471-0528.13429 PMID:26036300

Savona-Ventura, C., & Gatt, M. (2004). Embryonal risks in gestational diabetes mellitus. *Early Human Development*, *79*(1), 59–63. doi:10.1016/j.earlhumdev.2004.04.007 PMID:15449398

Selner, M. (2018). *Ectopic pregnancy*. Retrieved from https://www.healthline.com/health/pregnancy/ectopic-pregnancy

Setji, T. L., Brown, A. J., & Feinglos, M. N. (2005). Gestational Diabetes Mellitus. *Clinical Diabetes*, *23*(1), 17–24. doi:10.2337/diaclin.23.1.17

Sheehan, P. (2007). Hyperemesis gravidarum—assessment and management. *Australian Family Physician, 36*(9), 698–701.

Skipworth, R. (2011). A new clinical sign in ruptured ectopic pregnancy. *Lancet*, *378*(9809), e27. doi:10.1016/S0140-6736(11)61901-6 PMID:22177516

Slama, R., Bouyer, J., Windham, G., Fenster, L., Werwatz, A., & Swan, S. H. (2005). Influence of paternal age on the risk of spontaneous abortion. *American Journal of Epidemiology*, *161*(9), 816–823. doi:10.1093/aje/kwi097 PMID:15840613

Summers, A. (2012). Emergency management of hyperemesis gravidarum. *Emergency Nurse*, *20*(4), 24–28. doi:10.7748/en2012.07.20.4.24.c9206 PMID:22876404

Tabor, A., & Alfirevic, Z. (2010). Update on procedure-related risks for prenatal diagnosis techniques. *Fetal Diagnosis and Therapy*, *27*(1), 1–7. doi:10.1159/000271995 PMID:20051662

Tenore, J. L. (2000). Ectopic pregnancy. *American Family Physician*, *61*(4), 1080–1088. PMID:10706160

Tersigni, C., Castellani, R., de Waure, C., Fattorossi, A., De Spirito, M., Gasbarrini, A., Scambia, G., & Di Simone, N. (2014). Celiac disease and reproductive disorders: meta-analysis of epidemiologic associations and potential pathogenic mechanisms. *Human Reproduction Update, 20*(4), 582–593. doi:10.1093/humupd/dmu007

The Society of Obstetricians and Gynaecologists of Canada (SOGC). (2009). *Severe maternal morbidity in Canada*. Author.

Thompson, J. F., Roberts, C. L., Currie, M., & Ellwood, D. A. (2002). Prevalence and persistence of health problems after childbirth: Associations with parity and method of birth. *Birth (Berkeley, Calif.)*, *29*(2), 83–94. doi:10.1046/j.1523-536X.2002.00167.x PMID:12051189

Tieu, J., Shepherd, E., Middleton, P., & Crowther, C. A. (2017). Interconception care for women with a history of gestational diabetes for improving maternal and infant outcomes. *Cochrane Database of Systematic Reviews*, *8*, CD010211. doi:10.1002/14651858.CD010211.pub3 PMID:28836274

Toulis, K. A., Goulis, D. G., Kolibianakis, E. M., Venetis, C. A., Tarlatzis, B. C., & Papadimas, I. (2009). Risk of gestational diabetes mellitus in women with polycystic ovary syndrome: A systematic review and a meta-analysis. *Fertility and Sterility*, *92*(2), 667–677. doi:10.1016/j.fertnstert.2008.06.045 PMID:18710713

Tunçalp, O., Gülmezoglu, A. M., & Souza, J. P. (2010). Surgical procedures for evacuating incomplete miscarriage. *Cochrane Database of Systematic Reviews*, (9). doi:10.1002/14651858.CD001993.pub2 PMID:20824830

US National Library of Medicine (2013). Health problems in pregnancy. *Medline Plus*.

Vaiman, D. (2015). Genetic regulation of recurrent spontaneous abortion in humans. *Biomedical Journal*, *38*(1), 11–24. doi:10.4103/2319-4170.133777 PMID:25179715

Venners, S. A., Wang, X., Chen, C., Wang, L., Chen, D., Guang, W., Huang, A., Ryan, L., O'Connor, J., Lasley, B., Overstreet, J., Wilcox, A., & Xu, X. (2004). Paternal smoking and pregnancy loss: A prospective study using a biomarker of pregnancy. *American Journal of Epidemiology*, *159*(10), 993–1001. doi:10.1093/aje/kwh128 PMID:15128612

Viner, R. M., Coffey, C., Mathers, C., Bloem, P., Costello, A., Santelli, J., & Patton, G. C. (2011). 50-Year mortality trends in children and young people: A study of 50 low-income, middle-income, and high income countries. *Lancet*, *377*(9772), 1162–1174. doi:10.1016/S0140-6736(11)60106-2 PMID:21450338

Wahabi, H. A., Fayed, A. A., Esmaeil, S. A., & Al Zeidan, R. A. (2011). Progestogen for treating threatened miscarriage. Cochrane Database of Systematic Reviews, (12). doi:10.1002/14651858.CD005943.pub4

What are the symptoms of pregnancy loss/miscarriage? (2013). www.nichd.nih.gov

What are the treatments for pregnancy loss/miscarriage? (2013). www.nichd.nih.gov

Wilcox, A. J., Baird, D. D., & Weinberg, C. R. (1999). Time of implantation of the conceptus and loss of pregnancy. *The New England Journal of Medicine*, *340*(23), 1796–1799. doi:10.1056/NEJM199906103402304 PMID:10362823

World Health Organization. (2014). *Maternal Mortality*. Retrieved from www.who.int/reproductivehealth

Yamasmit, W., Chaithongwongwatthana, S., Tolosa, J. E., Limpongsanurak, S., Pereira, L., & Lumbiganon, P. (2015). Prophylactic oral betamimetics for reducing preterm birth in women with a twin pregnancy. *Cochrane Database of Systematic Reviews*, *12*(12). doi:10.1002/14651858.CD004733.pub4 PMID:26645888

Yin, Y. N., Li, X. L., Tao, T. J., Luo, B. R., & Liao, S. J. (2014). Physical activity during pregnancy and the risk of gestational diabetes mellitus: A systematic review and meta-analysis of randomized controlled trials. *British Journal of Sports Medicine*, *48*(4), 290–295. doi:10.1136/bjsports-2013-092596 PMID:24037671

Zhang, C., Bao, W., Rong, Y., Yang, H., Bowers, K., Yeung, E., & Kiely, M. (2013). Genetic variants and the risk of gestational diabetes mellitus: A systematic review. *Human Reproduction Update*, *19*(4), 376–390. doi:10.1093/humupd/dmt013 PMID:23690305

Zhang, J., Li, F., & Sheng, Q. (2008). Full-term abdominal pregnancy: A case report and review of the literature. *Gynecologic and Obstetric Investigation*, *65*(2), 139–141. doi:10.1159/000110015 PMID:17957101

Chapter 6
Labor Complications

ABSTRACT

A complication of labor is a problem that poses a risk to the mother's or baby's health that occurs during birth. There are also pregnancy complications; those are the health problems that occur in the pregnant woman or in the developing fetus before the onset of labour. Complications of birth may occur during labor or the delivery and can have serious repercussions for both mother and newborn. Some complications that women develop during pregnancy like preeclampsia (high blood pressure with protein in the urine) may lead to premature detachment of the placenta from the uterus (placental abruption) and problems in the newborn. Some other labor complications may sometimes develop spontaneously and unexpectedly. Hence, it becomes easier to anticipate such problems during pregnancy through regular antenatal check-up by a physician or a certified nurse/midwife. Thus, intrapartum care of women with a complicated labor and delivery is recommended to improve the chances of having a healthy baby and safe delivery.

KEY FACTS

- Worldwide, mostly as a result of unintended pregnancies, nearly 4.5 million adolescents undergo an abortion each year, with approximately 40 percent of abortions performed under unsafe conditions (Grimes et al, 2006).
- Nearly 10 percent of adolescent girls become mothers in low middle-income countries by the age of 16 years, with the highest rates in Sub-

DOI: 10.4018/978-1-7998-4357-3.ch006

Saharan Africa and South Central and Southeast Asia (World Health Organization, 2014).

- Unmarried adolescent mothers ' pregnancies are more likely to be unintended and likely to end in an induced abortion; coerced sex is reported by 10 percent of adolescent girls who first had sex before the age of 15 years, thus contributing to unwanted adolescent pregnancies, among many other negative effects (World Health Organization, 2014).
- Major complications related to obstetrics i.e. hemorrhage (33%), sepsis (21.7%) and eclampsia (7.5%), account for more than 75 percent of maternal deaths. These complications make a significant contribution to maternal mortality which are followed by non- hemorrhagic obstetric shock (5.6%), thrombo- embolism (5.6%) and obstructed labor (3.7%) (Dilpreet et al, 2007).
- In low middle-income countries, complications occurring during pregnancy and labour are the major causes of mortality among adolescent girls, aged 15 to 19 years, where almost all of the estimated three million abortions occur under unsafe conditions (Lopez et al, 2012).

INTRODUCTION

Parturition is a natural process that is simple. It can take a turn, however, making it "lethal" for any mother. "Normal delivery" is rightly said to be a retrospective diagnosis.

Maternal deaths are the tip of iceberg in most developing countries, which indicate the daily tragedies of women's lives. These also reflect how the worldwide poverty has been feminized. A woman dies every single minute. Every day nearly 1,400 women die which amounts to 0.6 million women dying annually. It is estimated that eighty percent of women die from pregnancy and childbirth complications and 99 percent of those deaths occur in Sub-Saharan Africa and South Asia (WHO/ UNICEF/ UNFPA, 2000). It was estimated by United Nations in 2003 that one out of every 55 women faces the risk of maternal mortality in India. Maternal mortality is, thus, a very difficult medical, social, emotional and hence medico-legal scenario prevalent in the third world countries (United Nations, 2003).

High-risk screening and proper antenatal, intra-natal and emergency obstetric care (EmOC) can prevent almost all major direct causes of maternal mortality. These include severe bleeding / hemorrhage (25%), infections / septicemia (13%), eclampsia (12%), obstructed labor (8%), complications of abortion (13%), other direct causes (8%) and indirect causes (20%) such as malaria, anemia, jaundice and other medical conditions that complicate or aggravate complications during pregnancy (Government of India, 2002). Hemorrhage, sepsis, eclampsia and obstructed labor account for 80 percent of all maternal deaths worldwide (Abou Zahr, 1998).

As a result of pregnancy, adolescents are more vulnerable to higher risk of complications and mortality as compared to their older counterparts. In Latin America, for example, the risk of maternal mortality is four-fold among young adolescents under 16 years of age as compared to older women in their twenties (World Health Organization, 2014). In terms of complications, anemia, malaria, HIV and other STI's, postpartum hemorrhage and mental disorders, such as depression, are associated with adolescent pregnancies (World Health Organization, 2014; Hodgkinson et al, 2010).

Pregnancy and delivery for adolescent girls, who have not yet completed their optimum body growth, expose them to multiple problems that are less common among adult women. An estimated 9 to 86 percent of women with obstetric fistula develop the condition as adolescents with traumatic and often lifelong negative consequences (Tebeu et al, 2012).

Low socioeconomic status, substance abuse and the likelihood of receiving low and/or inadequate prenatal care are all linked to adolescent pregnancies. The poor outcomes for adolescent mother's offspring are also well documented in the literature. These adverse outcomes include higher premature birth rates, babies with low birth weight and asphyxia leading to higher incidence of perinatal and neonatal mortality (Chen et al, 2007; World Health Organization, 2014; Lopez et al, 2012).

Sixteen million girls, aged 15 to 19 years, give birth each year which is approximately 11 percent of all births worldwide (World Health Organization, 2014); 95 percent of these births occur in low middle-income countries (LMIC's). There are significant regional differences; for example, adolescents giving births as a percentage of all births ranging from about 2 percent in China to 18 percent in Latin America and Caribbean which further rises to over 50 percent in Sub-Saharan Africa (World Health Organization, 2014).

The burden of complications during labor and delivery among adolescents' girls is higher than older woman. Many of the serious identified complications of pregnant mothers can be prevented. At national and local policies, the goals of safe motherhood and MDGs to be achieved must address to the needs of both women and young adolescents during labour and delivery. These must address the gaps in the prevention and various research programmes. To reduce the incidence of maternal and foetal morbidity and mortality rates, consistent and improved monitoring and appropriate interventions for the high-risk groups of pregnant women for maternal and fetal complications during labour and delivery are the key to achieve it(Hoque, 2011).

Pregnancy with Abortive Outcome

Regional differences, however, also exist; for example, 15 to 19-year-old adolescents account for 25 percent of all unsafe abortions in Africa but the proportion in Asia, Latin America and the Caribbean is much lower (Grimes et al, 2006). In Nigeria, up to 74 percent of all induced abortions which constitute approximately 60 percent of all gynecological hospital admissions occur among adolescents. In Tanzania, it was found that approximately half of the adolescent mothers seeking abortions were 17 years or younger in age (World Health Organization, 2007).

Researchers suggest that current contraceptive use prevents approximately 2, 72, 000 maternal mortalities per year and if current family planning needs were met, another 1, 04, 000 lives would not be lost (Ahmed et al, 2012), many of which would be adolescents' lives saved.

According to a report on abortion surveillance by the Centers for Disease Control and Prevention, 'Deaths of women associated with complications from abortion for the year 2015 are being assessed as part of the CDC's Pregnancy Mortality Surveillance System. Six women have been identified to have died as a result of complications from legal induced abortion in the year 2014, the most recent year for which data was available. However, unsafe abortion in other parts of the world is a leading cause of mortality among women having an unintended pregnancy. In a paper published in the year 2009, unsafe abortions are reported to be the reason of around 68,000 deaths among women every year (Murray, 2019).

The proportion of adolescent pregnancies that terminate into abortion has been found to vary widely across countries which have liberal abortion laws. The negative correlation between the rate of pregnancy and the proportion of pregnancies that end in abortion may reflect a planned larger proportion of pregnancies where rates are high. Alternatively, it might suggest that the constellation of forces that make it difficult for adolescents to prevent pregnancies such as very limited access to sexual and reproductive health services, including family planning etc. also make it difficult for them to terminate unplanned pregnancies.

Placenta Praevia

Placenta praevia is a condition when the placenta attaches itself inside the uterus but near or over the cervical opening (Merck Manuals Professional Edition, 2017*)*. Symptoms include vaginal bleeding in the second half of pregnancy *(Merck Manuals Professional Edition, 2017)*. The bleeding is bright red and tends not to be associated with pain *(*Merck Manuals Professional Edition, 2017). *It is classified as a complication of pregnancy (*Merck Manuals Professional Edition, 2017).

It is not known what exactly causes placenta praevia. It is hypothesized to be associated with abnormal endometrial vascularization which is usually due to scarring or atrophy from earlier trauma, surgery or infection. Such factors can hinder the lower segment's differential growth, leading to less upward shift in the position of placenta with the advancement of the pregnancy (Dashe et al, 2002).

Epidemiology

The condition was first described in 1685 by Paul Portal *(Baskett et al, 2014)*. Placenta praevia occurs approximately in one of every 200 births globally *(Cresswell et al, 2013)*. It has been suggested that rates of placenta praevia are increasing due to an increased rate of Caesarian section *(Miller et al, 1997)*.

Reasons for regional variation may include ethnicity and diet *(Cresswell et al, 2013)*. Placenta praevia affects approximately 0.5 percent of total pregnancies *(Cresswell et al, 2013)*. After four cesarean sections, however, it affects 10 percent of total pregnancies *(Allahdin et al, 2011)*. Rates of the condition have increased over the late 20th century and early 21st century *(Palacios-Jaraquemada, 2013)*.

Risk Factors

Risk factors of placenta praevia include pregnancy at an older age and smoking as well as prior cesarean section, labor induction or termination of pregnancy (Palacios-Jaraquemada, 2013; Allahdin et al, 2011).

Women, who are younger than 20 years of age, are at a higher risk and women older than 35 years of age are at an increasing risk, as they get older. Women, who have had previous pregnancies (multiparity), especially a large number of closely spaced pregnancies, are also at a higher risk due to the uterine damage of the mother (Brinsden and Murray, 2006).

Other compounding factors could be previous history of placenta previa (recurrence rate is 4 to 8 percent) (Kendrick and Hazel Everitt, 2005), caesarean delivery (Weerasekera, 2000), myomectomy (Brinsden et al, 2006) or endometrium damage caused by D&C (Kendrick and Hazel Everitt, 2005). Women with a large placenta from twins or erythroblastosis are also at a higher risk. Alcohol use during pregnancy is also listed as a risk factor of placenta praevia (Aliyu et al, 2011). Smoking during pregnancy (Arulkumaran, 2009) and cocaine use during pregnancy could also be the contributing factors (Handler et al, 1991; Kistin et al, 1996).

Race is, however, a controversial risk factor. Some studies reveal higher risk of placenta previa among certain races while others studies reveal no racial differences. Placenta previa itself poses a risk of placenta accreta.

Symptoms

There is painless, bright red vaginal bleeding in women with placenta previa which commonly occurs around 32 weeks of gestation. However, it can be as early or as late as the mid-trimester (*Callander et al, 2004)*. More than half of women affected by placenta praevia (51.6 percent) have bleeding before the delivery (Fan et al, 2017). With an increase as the area of placental separation, the bleeding which often starts mildly may increase. Bleeding after 24 weeks of gestation should be suspected for placenta praevia. In about 22 percent of those affected with placenta praevia, bleeding occurs after delivery (*Fan et al, 2017)*. Women may also present as a case of failure of engagement of foetal head (*Brinsden and Murray, 2006)*.

Treatment

For women who are pregnant for less than 36 weeks of gestation with only a small amount of bleeding, recommendations include bed rest and avoiding any sexual activity. Cäsarean-section is generally recommended for those after 36 weeks of pregnancy or with a significant amount of bleeding. Corticosteroids may be given to women with less than 36 weeks of pregnancy to facilitate the development of the baby's lungs. Complications occurring during early pregnancy usually resolve by themselves. Diagnosis is through ultrasonography screening (*Merck Manuals Professional Edition, 2017).*

Complications

Complications associated with placenta praevia may include placenta accreta, dangerously low blood pressure or bleeding after delivery (Fan et al, 2017; *Allahdin et al, 2011).* Placenta praevia may lead to ante-partum and post-partum hemorrhage, malpresentation and abnormal placentation. The risk of puerperal sepsis and postpartum hemorrhage is increasingly posed by placenta previa due to lower segment, to which the placenta is attached, contracting less during post-delivery. Complications for the baby may include fetal growth restriction (Intra Uterine Growth Retardation (IUGR) up to15 percent incidence), hypoxia, premature delivery and death (*Kendrick and Hazel Everitt, 2005).*

Breech Presentation

Sometimes, baby is in an unusual presentation i.e. breech (buttocks first) or transverse (lying horizontally across the womb). A baby is in a breech position if its feet are positioned to be delivered before the delivery of the head. According to the APA, its incidence is about 4 percent of full-term births.

A baby with breech presentation may be lying in one of these three positions, known as extended (frank), flexed (complete) or footling (incomplete). The hips are flexed with an extended breech position, knees extended and the feet are by the baby's head. With this type of breech, a vaginal delivery is most likely to occur. Hips and knees are flexed in a flexed breech, the feet above the buttocks and a vaginal birth in this position may also be possible. In a footling breech, the hips are stretched with the feet below the baby's buttocks, thereby reducing the likelihood of vaginal delivery occurring normally.

At 32 weeks of gestation, almost 15 percent of the babies are breech. With time, most of them turn and just 3 to 4 percent remain breech at full term gestation. Breech labors and births are usually more difficult. In such a position, there is a procedure to turn the baby. The procedure is called External Cephalic Version (ECV) and is usually offered at 37 weeks of gestation if the baby is still in a breech position. In this procedure, the lower part of stomach is pressed to raise the bottom of the baby out of the pelvis. Pressure is applied to rotate the baby to make its head down. This procedure is uncomfortable and thus requires medication to relax the uterus of the mother. A scanning is helpful for guidance during the procedure.

The rate of success in the External Cephalic Versions (ECV's) is often over 40 percent. There can be complications such as bleeding behind the placenta and uterine rupture but chances are rare. If an External Cephalic Version (ECV) is unsuccessful, it is advisable to deliver in a hospital for the vaginal birth. In some cases, the position of a breech baby is likely to make the vaginal delivery difficult and then Caesarean delivery is advised.

However, if the breech presentation is diagnosed during labour, ECV can still be done, though it has lower success rate. Sometimes, it may not be possible to offer ECV in labour if the water bag has already ruptured and the labour has advanced or if there is no one to do the procedure.

Majority of babies born in breech position are usually healthy. However, the doctors recommend not going ahead with a vaginal birth in case the baby shows the signs of distress or the baby is too big to pass the birth canal safely. If the doctor finds a few weeks before delivery that the baby is in the breech position, it is possible to change the baby's position. Most doctors recommend a cesarean delivery if the baby is still in the breech position when labour begins.

Cesarean Delivery

Caesarean section is an effective strategy to save the lives of both mother and the newborn. The available evidence indicates that caesarean section rates higher than 10 percent of the population level are not linked with the decreases in maternal and neonatal mortality rates. Hence, this may not be required to achieve the objective of lowering the maternal and neonatal mortality rates (WHO, 2015). The rate of Caesarean section is defined as a percentage drawn by dividing the number of caesarean sections over the total number of live births in a duration which is usually one year.

The possibilities of death from a cesarean section are still rare in developed countries but it is a little higher than a vaginal delivery. A 2008 study published in the American Journal of Obstetrics and Gynecology reported that maternal mortality for C-sections is 2.2 per 100,000 livebirths and for vaginal births, it is 0.2 per 100,000 livebirths (Clark et al, 2008). Another research published in 2010 revealed that if a C-section is elective and performed without medical advice, the risks involved are greater than the vaginal delivery.

The reason why a Cesarean section has a higher risk rate is that it is a surgery and every surgery involves some risk. Some complications may arise from a C-section that may lead to maternal death. These include infection, blood clots, anesthesia reactions, blood loss or injury to some other organs which may occur during the surgery.

However, C-sections save lives too are an important thing to be kept under consideration. Under certain conditions, a C-section is the best option. Whenever required, a cesarean section reduces the chances of maternal death as well as neonatal death and makes the delivery safe for both mother as well as the child.

Over the past three decades, World Health Organization (WHO) has proposed a caesarean section rate of 10 to 15 percent which was used as a threshold (Appropriate technology for birth, 1985), despite the lack of concrete supporting evidence for that statement. Several ecological studies analyzed the association between mode of delivery and maternal, neonatal and infant mortality rates. These studies also identified an inflection point below which a strong association exists between cäsarean section rates and mortality rates (Betran et al, 2007; Ye et al, 2014; Jurdi and Khawaja, 2004; McClure et al, 2007; Althabe et al, 2006; Belizan et al, 1999; Silva et al, 2010; Volpe, 2011; Zizza et al, 2011).

Worldwide, Caesarean section rates have risen substantially since 1980's (Gibbons et al, 2012; Betran et al, 2007: Robson, 2001; Ye et al, 2014). In some countries, this rate has increased several-fold since the year 1985 when World Health Organization (WHO) suggested a caesarean section rate of 10 to 15 percent as the upper limit at the population level (Appropriate technology for birth, 1985). Though, the rate is still below 10 percent in some under-developed countries, mostly in Africa yet the majority of the countries have super ceded this recommendation. However, some countries have exceeded it by a huge margin (Gibbons et al, 2012; Betran et al, 2007; Ye et al, 2014).

The reasons for such a dramatic increase in the caesarean section rate are multi-factorial, including medical as well as non-medical reasons (Robson, 2001; Gibbons et al, 2012; Zhang et al, 2010). It was suggested that non-medical factors such as social, cultural or unequal accessibility to health care services, as well as patterns / styles of clinical practice, could have contributed significantly to the wide variations in the rates of caesarean section across various nations (Gibbons et al, 2010; Betran et al, 2007; Gibbons et al, 2012; Zhang et al, 2010; Fioretti et al, 2015; Torloni et al, 2013; Torloni et al, 2014). On the other side, it can be assumed that the rates of the caesarean section under medical advice, which is associated with the lowest maternal and neonatal mortality, should differ less between countries if the same indications for the Caesarean section were applied across all countries (Ye et al, 2014; Joffe et al, 1994).

Caesarean section rates have risen over the last 12 years in most countries around the world. More developed countries had higher baselines and higher rises in Caesarean section rates in absolute terms than the least and less developed countries; however, the maternal and neonatal mortality rates in those countries only slightly changed during the corresponding period. On the contrary, Caesarean section rates showed the most relative rise in the least developed countries. Maternal and neonatal mortality rates decreased substantially, with a small absolute increase in the rate of Caesarean section in the least developed countries (Ye et al, 2015).

The significant and negative relationship between Caesarean section rates and mortality rates was only found when the Caesarean section rate was below 5 to 10 percent. The association was less pronounced after adjustment for the Human Development Index (HDI), i.e. the crude association appears to be explained mainly by socio-economic conditions. Furthermore, the analysis reveals that a caesarean section rate above 10 percent at population level may not be significantly correlated with the rates of maternal and neonatal mortality (Ye et al, 2015).

It was observed that higher rates of caesarean section had been linked with lower rates of maternal and infant mortality until a particular point, called the inflection point, above which rates of caesarean section were not significantly associated with these results. This inflection point, as a Caesarean section rate, was deemed necessary from a medical point of view to minimize mortality. However, the findings and interpretations of results in these studies were restricted by the cross-sectional nature of the ecological data. Further, most of these studies had not monitored the socio-economic conditions that had a major impact on both the availability of caesarean section and maternal and perinatal mortality, thereby confounding the association between caesarean section rates and their adverse results (Betran et al, 2007; Jurdi and Khawaja, 2004; McClure et al, 2007; Silva et al, 2010; Volpe, 2011; Zizza et al, 2011).

After adjusting for socio-economic conditions, the negative association found between Caesarean section rates and neonatal mortality rates was statistically non-significant. However, an inflection point of Caesarean section rate based on the adjusted models was not demonstrated (Althabe et al, 2006).

Another study supported the World Health Organization's reference and suggested a Caesarean section rate at 10 to 15 percent based on its association with mortality outcomes, after adjusting for Gross Domestic Product (GDP) and Human Development Index (HDI) (Ye et al, 2014). The analysis further revealed that after adjusting for socio-economic development, a substantially less pronounced association and an even lower threshold for a significant association between rates of Caesarean section and rates of maternal and neonatal mortality at the population level had been suggested (Ye et al, 2014).

The study revealed that socio-economic status strongly influenced the association between caesarean section rates and mortality rates. Socio-economic differences can, therefore, be a significant factor to explain most of the crude association between the rate of Caesarean section and mortality outcomes. The significant and negative association between Caesarean section rate and mortality was observed, after adjustment for the Human Development Index (HDI), when the Caesarean section rate was below 10 per cent. The inflection point appears below other investigators ' reported numbers (Ye et al, 2014; McClure et al, 2007; Silva et al, 2010; Volpe, 2011; confound the association between Caesarean section rates and adverse outcomes (Betran et al, 2007; Jurdi and Khawaja, 2004; McClure et al, 2007; Silva et al, 2010; Volpe, 2011; Zizza et al, 2011).

A systematic review of these ecological studies concluded that this infliction point ranged between 9 to 16 percent. There was no longer any association between Caesarean section rates and maternal or infant mortality rates at Caesarean section rates above this threshold (Betran et al, 2015). One of these studies also reported that even after making adjustments for the gross national income, there was a negative association between Caesarean section rates and maternal mortality rates, the proportion of skilled attendance deliveries and the proportion of literate populations in low-income countries (Althabe et al, 2006).

In the United States, most of the maternal deaths cannot be prevented and happen to women who start their pregnancy without significant mortality risk factors. Though the observations with regard to the association between cesarean delivery and maternal mortality are confirmed yet a much smaller causative relationship existed between the two. The data suggested that the excessive risk of mortality due to cesarean delivery can be virtually eliminated with an appropriate prophylaxis of the universal thrombo-embolism. The overall risk of mortality attributable to this prophylaxis would be less than 1 per 100,000 live-births. Thus, with the given potential for bleeding complications using neuraxial anesthesia methods which are commonly used in a cesarean delivery, it is recommended to use the process of implementing a policy of universal pneumatic compression device for all women who undergo a cesarean delivery in the health care system (Clark et al, 2008).

Low Birth weight

A substantial proportion of teen births are intended in developing countries where many women still marry early (Kothari et al, 2012). However, policy and public health relevance is of great significance for reducing even the intended pregnancies among young women in low resource settings due to the risks involved in them. The risk of pregnancy associated death is about a third higher among 15 to 19-year young adolescent mothers as compared to 20 to 24 year old mother (Nove et al, 2012). It also suggests that young adolescent mothers are more likely to experience obstructed labor, fistula and premature delivery and also likely to give birth to babies with low birth weight as compared to their older counterparts (UNFPA, 2013).

World Health organization has defined Low birth weight (LBW) as a birth weight of an infant of 2,499 gm or less, regardless of the age of gestation (ICD-10). Low birth weight of newborn is either due to preterm birth i.e. a low gestational age at birth which is usually defined as less than 37 weeks of gestation or an infant being small for its gestational age i.e. an impaired prenatal growth rate or a combination of two.

The *Agency for Healthcare Research and Quality (AHRQ)* undertook a study and reported that approximately 6.1 percent (231,900) of the 3.8 million births that occurred in the United States of America in 2011 were diagnosed with low birth weight (< 2,500 gms). About 49,300 newborns had birth weight less than 1,500 grams (VLBW) which constituted 1.3 per cent of total births. Children with low birth weight were predisposed to an increased risk of developing neonatal infections (Kowlessar et al, 2013).

Generally, the mother's risk factors that can contribute to low birth weight of infants include mother's young age, multiple pregnancies, previous history of infants with low birth weight, poor nutrition, heart disease or hypertension, untreated celiac disease, drug addiction, alcohol abuse as well as an inadequate prenatal care. However, the environmental risk factors are smoking, lead exposure and other types of lead pollution that can contribute to newborn's low birth weight (Tersigni et al, 2014; Saccone et al, 2015).

Infants are generally born with low weight due to poor nutrition of mother or the use of cigarettes, alcohol or drugs consumed during pregnancy. Low birth weight babies are at an increased risk of respiratory infections, learning disabilities, heart infections and blindness. The baby may require a few months of hospitalization after birth (Andrew et al, 2008; Norton, 2005).

In the developing countries, low birth weight contributes to 60 to 80 percent of infant mortality rates. Low birth weight leading to infant mortality is usually caused by other medical conditions such as premature birth, poor maternal nutritional status, lack of prenatal care, any maternal disease during pregnancy and an unhygienic environment at home (Andrew et al, 2008; Norton, 2005).

Low birth weight is intimately related to foetal and perinatal mortality and morbidity, followed by impaired growth and inhibited cognitive development and chronic diseases in later life. The proportion of babies with low birth weight at population level is an indicator of a multifaceted public health problem that includes long-term maternal malnutrition, poor health, hard work and poor pregnancy health care. Individually, low birth weight is an important predictor of neonatal health and survival and is linked with an increased risk of infant and child mortality (Stevens-Simons and Orleans, 1999).

CONCLUSION

World Health Organization, in the year 1997, defined normal birth as 'spontaneous in onset, low risk at the onset of labour and remaining so throughout labour and delivery. An infant is born in the vertex position spontaneously between 37 to 42 complete weeks of gestation. After birth, both the mother and newborn are in good condition' (WHO, 1997). However, the Intrapartum care of women with a complicated labour and delivery is required for cases such as malpresentation, preterm labour, operative vaginal delivery, maternal medical/obstetric disorders, hemorrhage etc. It is also important to ensure that someone with midwifery training is present at every delivery; in the developing countries, only 51 percent of all births are professionally attended (Ross et al, 1999).

Four factors important in determining the satisfaction of a woman with her child birth experience include her personal expectations, the amount of support she receives, the quality of caregiver-patient relationship i.e. respect, communication and continuity of care and her involvement in decision making with regard to child birth, which make child bearing a pleasant experience.

REFERENCES

Abou Zahr, C. (1998). Maternal mortality overview. In C. J. L. Murrary & A. D. Lopez (Eds.), *Health dimensions of sex and reproduction* (Vol. 111, p. 64). World Health Organization.

Ahmed, S., Li, Q., Liu, L., & Tsui, A. O. (2012). Maternal deaths averted by contraceptive use: An analysis of 172 countries. *Lancet*, *380*(9837), 111–125. doi:10.1016/S0140-6736(12)60478-4 PMID:22784531

Aliyu, M. H., Lynch, O., Nana, P. N., Alio, A. P., Wilson, R. E., Marty, P. J., Zoorob, R., & Salihu, H. M. (2011). Alcohol consumption during pregnancy and risk of placental abruption and placenta previa. *Maternal and Child Health Journal*, *15*(5), 670–676. doi:10.100710995-010-0615-6 PMID:20437196

Allahdin, S., Voigt, S., & Htwe, T. T. (2011). Management of placenta praevia and accrete. *Journal of Obstetrics & Gynaecology*, *31*(1), 1–6. doi:10.3109/01443615.2010.532248 PMID:21280984

Althabe, F., Sosa, C., Belizan, J. M., Gibbons, L., Jacquerioz, F., & Bergel, E. (2006). Cesarean section rates and maternal and neonatal mortality in low-,medium- and high-income countries: An ecological study. *Birth (Berkeley, Calif.)*, *33*(4), 270–277. doi:10.1111/j.1523-536X.2006.00118.x PMID:17150064

Andrew, K. M., Brouillette, D. B., & Brouillette, R. T. (2008). Mortality, Infant. Encyclopedia of infant and early childhood development, 343-359.

Appropriate technology for birth. (1985). *Lancet*, *2*, 436–7.

Arulkumaran. (2009). *Best practice in labour and delivery* (3rd ed.). Cambridge, UK: Cambridge University Press.

Baskett, T. F., Calder, A. A., & Arulkumaran, S. (2014). *Munro Kerr's Operative Obstetrics E-Book*. Elsevier Health Sciences.

Belizan, J. M., Althabe, F., Barros, F. C., Alexander, S., Showalter, E., Griffin, A., Castro, A., & Bastian, H. (1999). Rates and implications of caesarean sections in Latin America: An ecological study. *British Medical Journal*, *319*(7222), 1397–1400. doi:10.1136/bmj.319.7222.1397 PMID:10574855

Betran, A. P., Merialdi, M., Lauer, J. A., Bing-Shun, W., Thomas, J., Van Look, P., & Wagner, M. (2007). Rates of caesarean section: Analysis of global, regional and national estimates. *Paediatric and Perinatal Epidemiology*, *21*(2), 98–113. doi:10.1111/j.1365-3016.2007.00786.x PMID:17302638

Betran, A. P., Torloni, M. R., Zhang, J., Ye, J., Mikolajczyk, R., Deneux-Tharaux, C., Oladapo, O. T., Souza, J. P., Tunçalp, Ö., Vogel, J. P., & Gülmezoglu, A. M. (2015). What is the optimal rate of caesarean section at population level? A systematic review of ecologic studies. *Reproductive Health*, *12*(1), 57. doi:10.118612978-015-0043-6 PMID:26093498

Blanc, A. K., Tsui, A. O., Croft, T. N., & Trevitt, J. L. (2009). Patterns and trends in adolescents' contraceptive use and discontinuation in developing countries and comparisons with adult women. *International Perspectives on Sexual and Reproductive Health*, *35*(2), 63–71. doi:10.1363/3506309 PMID:19620090

Blot, M. (2018). *The DAY-BY-DAY Pregnancy Book*. Penguin Random House.

Brinsden, J. C., & Murray, L. M. (2006). *Oxford handbook of clinical specialties* (7th ed.). Oxford University Press.

Callander, K. P. (2004). Obstetrics illustrated (6th ed.). Edinburgh, UK: Churchill Livingstone.

Chandra-Mouli, V., McCarraher, D. R., Phillips, S. J., Williamson, N. E., & Hainsworth, G. (2014). Contraception for adolescents in low and middle income countries: Needs, barriers and access. *Reproductive Health*, *11*(1), 1. doi:10.1186/1742-4755-11-1 PMID:24383405

Chen, X. K., Wen, S. W., Fleming, N., Demissie, K., Rhoads, G. G., & Walker, M. (2007). Teenage pregnancy and adverse birth outcomes: A large population based retrospective cohort study. *International Journal of Epidemiology*, *36*(2), 368–373. doi:10.1093/ije/dyl284 PMID:17213208

Clark, S. L., Belfort, M.A., Dildy, G.A., Herbst, M.A., Meyers, J.A., & Hankins, G.D. (2008). Maternal death in the 21st century: causes, prevention and relationship to cesarean delivery. *American Journal of Obstetrics and Gynecology, 199*(1). doi:10.1016/j.ajog.2008.03.007

Cresswell, J.A., Ronsmans, C., Calvert, C. & Filippi, V. (2013). Prevalence of placenta praevia by world region: A systematic review and meta-analysis. *Tropical Medicine and International Health (TM & IH), 18*(6), 712–24. doi:10.1111/tmi.12100

Dashe, J. S., McIntire, D. D., Ramus, R. M., Santos-Ramos, R., & Twickler, D. M. (2002). Persistence of placenta previa according to gestational age at ultrasound detection. *Obstetrics and Gynecology, 99*(5 Pt 1), 692–697. doi:10.10160029-7844(02)01935-x PMID:11978274

Dilpreet, K., Vaneet, K., & Veronica, I. Y. (2007). Alarmingly High Maternal Mortality in 21st Century. *JK Science, 9*(3), 123–126.

Fan, D., Wu, S., Liu, L., Xia, Q., Wang, W., Guo, X., & Liu, Z. (2017). Prevalence of antepartum hemorrhage in women with placenta previa: A systematic review and meta-analysis. *Scientific Reports, 7*(1), 40320. doi:10.1038rep40320 PMID:28067303

Fan, D., Xia, Q., Liu, L., Wu, S., Tian, G., Wang, W., Wu, S., Guo, X., & Liu, Z. (2017). The Incidence of Postpartum Hemorrhage in Pregnant Women with Placenta Previa: A Systematic Review and Meta-Analysis. *PLoS One, 12*(1), e0170194. doi:10.1371/journal.pone.0170194 PMID:28107460

Fioretti, B., Reiter, M., Betran, A., & Torloni, M. (2015). Googling caesarean section: A survey on the quality of the information available on the Internet. *British Journal of Obstetrics and Gynaecology, 122*(5), 731–739. doi:10.1111/1471-0528.13081 PMID:25209160

Govt of India. (2002). *Annual Report 2001-2002.* Ministry of Health and Family Welfare.

Gibbons, L., Belizan, J.M., Lauer, J.A., Betran, A.P., Merialdi, M., & Althabe, F. (2010). *The Global Numbers and Costs of Additionally Needed and Unnecessary Caesarean Sections Performed per Year: Overuse as a Barrier to Universal Coverage.* World Health Report Background Paper, No 30.

Gibbons, L., Belizan, J. M., Lauer, J. A., Betran, A. P., Merialdi, M., & Althabe, F. (2012). Inequities in the use of cesarean section deliveries in the world. *American Journal of Obstetrics and Gynecology, 206*(4), 331.e1–331.e19. doi:10.1016/j.ajog.2012.02.026 PMID:22464076

Grimes, D. A., Benson, J., Singh, S., Romero, M., Ganatra, B., Okonofua, F. E., & Shah, I. H. (2006). Unsafe abortion: The preventable pandemic. *Lancet*, *368*(9550), 1908–1919. doi:10.1016/S0140-6736(06)69481-6 PMID:17126724

Handler, A., Kistin, N., Davis, F., & Ferré, C. (1991). Cocaine use during pregnancy: Perinatal outcomes. *American Journal of Epidemiology*, *133*(8), 818–825. doi:10.1093/oxfordjournals.aje.a115961 PMID:2021149

Hoque, M. (2011). *Incidence of Obstetric and Foetal Complications during Labor and Delivery at a Community Health Centre*. Midwives Obstetric Unit of Durban.

Hodgkinson, S. C., Colantuoni, E., Roberts, D., Berg-Cross, L., & Belcher, H. M. (2010). Depressive symptoms and birth outcomes among pregnant teenagers. *Journal of Pediatric and Adolescent Gynecology*, *23*(1), 16–22. doi:10.1016/j.jpag.2009.04.006 PMID:19679498

International Planned Parenthood Federation (IPPF). (2010). *Facts on the sexual and reproductive health of adolescent women in the developing world*. New York: Guttmacher Institute. https://www.guttmacher.org/pubs/FB-Adolescents-SRH.pdf

Jaraquemada, J. M. (2013). Caesarean section in cases of placenta praevia and accrete. *Best Practice & Research. Clinical Obstetrics & Gynaecology*, *27*(2), 221–232. doi:10.1016/j.bpobgyn.2012.10.003 PMID:23127895

Joffe, M., Chapple, J., Paterson, C., & Beard, R. W. (1994). What is the optimal caesarean section rate? An outcome based study of existing variation. *Journal of Epidemiology and Community Health*, *48*(4), 406–411. doi:10.1136/jech.48.4.406 PMID:7964342

Jurdi, R., & Khawaja, M. (2004). Caesarean section rates in the Arab region: A cross-national study. *Health Policy and Planning*, *19*(2), 101–110. doi:10.1093/heapol/czh012 PMID:14982888

Kothari, M. T., Wang, S., & Head, S. (2012). *Trends in adolescent reproductive and sexual behaviors. Demographic and Health Surveys Comparative Reports No. 29*. ICF International.

Kendrick, C. S., & Hazel Everitt, T. (2005). *Oxford handbook of general practice* (2nd ed.). Oxford University Press.

Kistin, N., Handler, A., Davis, F., & Ferre, C. (1996). Cocaine and cigarettes: A comparison of risks. *Paediatric and Perinatal Epidemiology, 10*(3), 269–278. doi:10.1111/j.1365-3016.1996.tb00050.x PMID:8822770

Kowlessar, N. M., Jiang, H. J., & Steiner, C. (2013). *Hospital Stays for Newborns, 2011. HCUP Statistical Brief# 163. Agency for Healthcare Research and Quality*. AHRQ.

Lopez, L. M., Hiller, J. E., & Grimes, D. A. (2012). Education for contraceptive use by women after childbirth. *Cochrane Database of Systematic Reviews, 8*, CD001863. PMID:22895923

McClure, E. M., Goldenberg, R. L., & Bann, C. M. (2007). Maternal mortality, stillbirth and measures of obstetric care in developing and developed countries. *International Journal of Gynaecology and Obstetrics: the Official Organ of the International Federation of Gynaecology and Obstetrics, 96*(2), 139–146. doi:10.1016/j.ijgo.2006.10.010 PMID:17274999

Merck Manuals Professional Edition. (2017). *Placenta Previa – Gynecology and Obstetrics – Merck Manuals Professional Edition*. Author.

Miller, D. A., Chollet, J. A., & Goodwin, T. M. (1997). Clinical risk factors for placenta previa-placenta accreta. *American Journal of Obstetrics and Gynecology, 177*(1), 210–214. doi:10.1016/S0002-9378(97)70463-0 PMID:9240608

Murray Donna, R. N. (2019). *Maternal Mortality Rate, Causes, and Prevention*. https://www.verywellfamily.com/maternal-mortality-rate-causes-and-prevention-4163653Palacios-

Norton, M. (2005). New evidence on birth spacing: Promising findings for improving newborn, infant, child and maternal health. *International Journal of Gynaecology and Obstetrics: the Official Organ of the International Federation of Gynaecology and Obstetrics, 89*, S1–S6. doi:10.1016/j.ijgo.2004.12.012 PMID:15820364

Nove, A., Matthews, Z. & Neal, S. (2012). Maternal mortality in adolescents compared with women of other ages: Evidence from 144 countries. *The Lancet Global Health, 2*, e155-e64.

Robson, M. S. (2001). Can we reduce the caesarean section rate? *Best Practice & Research. Clinical Obstetrics & Gynaecology, 15*(1), 179–194. doi:10.1053/beog.2000.0156 PMID:11359322

Ross, G. (2006). Gestational diabetes. *Australian Family Physician, 35*(6), 392–396. PMID:16751853

Saccone, G., Berghella, G., Sarno, L., Maruotti, G. M., Cetin, I., Greco, L., Khashan, A. S., McCarthy, F., Martinelli, D., Fortunato, F., & Martinelli, P. (2015). Coeilac diseases and obstetric complications: A systematic review and meta-analysis. *American Journal of Obstetrics and Gynecology, 214*(2), 225–234. doi:10.1016/j.ajog.2015.09.080 PMID:26432464

Silva, A. A., Silva, L. M., Barbieri, M. A., Bettiol, H., Carvalho, L. M., Ribeiro, V. S., & Goldani, M. Z. (2010). The epidemiologic paradox of low birth weight in Brazil. *Revista de Saude Publica, 44*(5), 767–775. doi:10.1590/S0034-89102010005000033 PMID:20835496

Singh, S., & Darroch, J. E. (2012). *Adding it up: Costs and benefits of contraceptive service. Estimates for 2012*. Guttmacher Institute and UNFPA. http://www. guttmacher.org/pubs/AIU-2012-estimates.pdf

Stevens-Simons, C., & Orleans, M. (1999). Low birth weight prevention programs: The enigma of failure. *Birth (Berkeley, Calif.), 26*(3), 184–191. doi:10.1046/j.1523-536x.1999.00184.x PMID:10655819

Tebeu, P. M., Fomulu, J. N., Khaddaj, S., de Bernis, L., Delvaux, T., & Rochat, C. H. (2012). Risk factors for obstetric fistula: A clinical review. *International Urogynecology Journal and Pelvic Floor Dysfunction, 23*(4), 387–394. doi:10.100700192-011-1622-x PMID:22143450

Tersigni, C., Castellani, R., de Waure, C., Fattorossi, A., De Spirito, M., Gasbarrini, A., Scambia, G., & Di Simone, N. (2014). Coeilac diseases and reproductive disorders: Meta-analysis of epidemiologic associations and potential pathogenic mechanisms. *Human Reproduction Update, 20*(4), 582–593. doi:10.1093/humupd/dmu007 PMID:24619876

Torloni, M. R., Betran, A. P., Montilla, P., Scolaro, E., Seuc, A., Mazzoni, A., Althabe, F., Merzagora, F., Donzelli, G. P., & Merialdi, M. (2013). Do Italian women prefer cesarean section? Results from a survey on mode of delivery preferences. *BoiMed Central Pregnancy and Childbirth, 13*(1), 78. doi:10.1186/1471-2393-13-78 PMID:23530472

Torloni, M. R., Campos Mansilla, B., Merialdi, M., & Betran, A. P. (2014). What do popular Spanish women's magazines say about caesarean section? A 21-year survey. *British Journal of Obstetrics and Gynaecology, 121*(5), 548–555. doi:10.1111/1471-0528.12513 PMID:24467797

UNFPA. (2013). *Motherhood in childhood: Facing the challenge of adolescent pregnancy: The State of World Population 2013*. United Nations Population Fund.

United Nations. (2003). *Convention on the Rights of the Child. General Comment No. 4. Adolescent health and development in the context of the Convention on the Rights of the Child*. CRC/GC/2003/4. http://daccess-dds-ny.un.org/doc/UNDOC/GEN/G03/427/24/PDF/G0342724.pdf?OpenElement

United Nations. (2013). *Adolescent fertility since the International Conference on Population and Development (ICPD) in Cairo*. United Nations.

Volpe, F. M. (2011). Correlation of Cesarean rates to maternal and infant mortality rates: An ecologic study of official international data. *Revista Panamericana de Salud Pública, 29*(5), 303–308. doi:10.1590/S1020-49892011000500001 PMID:21709933

Weerasekera, D. S. (2000). Placenta previa and scarred uterus— An obstetrician's dilemma. *Journal of Obstetrics & Gynaecology, 20*(5), 484–485. doi:10.1080/014436100434659 PMID:15512632

World Health Organization. (1997). Care in normal birth: A practical guide. Technical Working Group, World Health Organization. *Birth (Berkeley, Calif.), 24*(2), 121–123. doi:10.1111/j.1523-536X.1997.tb00352.x PMID:9271979

World Health Organization. (2007). *Adolescent pregnancy: unmet needs and undone deeds: A review of the literature and programmes*. WHO.

World Health Organization. (2015). *WHO statement on caesarean section rates*. Retrieved from https://www.who.int/reproductivehealth/publications/maternal_perinatal_health/cs-statement/en/

World Health Organization. (2014a). *Maternal, newborn, child and adolescent health. Adolescent pregnancy.* Retrieved from https://www.who.int/maternal_child_adolescent/topics/maternal/adolescent_pregnancy/en/. Accessed October 24, 2014.

World Health Organization. (2014b). *Adolescent pregnancy. Fact sheet No. 364*. https://www.who.int/mediacentre/factsheets/fs364/en/

Ye, J., Betran, A. P., Guerrero Vela, M., Souza, J. P., & Zhang, J. (2014). Searching for the optimal rate of medically necessary cesarean delivery. *Birth (Berkeley, Calif.), 41*(3), 237–244. doi:10.1111/birt.12104 PMID:24720614

Ye, J., Zhang, J., Mikolajczyk, R., Torloni, M. R., Gülmezoglu, A. M., & Betran, A. P. (2016). Association between rates of caesarean section and maternal and neonatal mortality in the 21st century: A worldwide population-based ecological study with longitudinal data. *British Journal of Obstetrics and Gynaecology*, *123*(5), 745–753. doi:10.1111/1471-0528.13592 PMID:26331389

Zhang, J., Troendle, J., Reddy, U.M., Laughon, S.K., Branch, D.W. & Burkman, R. (2010). Contemporary cesarean delivery practice in the United States. *American Journal of Obstetrics and Gynecology, 203*, 326.e1–.e10.

Zizza, A., Tinelli, A., Malvasi, A., Barbone, E., Stark, M., & De Donno, A. (2011). Caesarean section in the world: Anew ecological approach. *Journal of Preventive Medicine and Hygiene*, *52*, 161–173. PMID:22442920

Chapter 7
Puerperal Disorders

ABSTRACT

Unfortunately, the complexities of human pregnancy and birth make it a risky endeavor. The most vulnerable time for maternal death is the post-partum period during which 60% deaths and 65% deaths are reported. Around 62.3% deaths are estimated to occur in post-partum period. Unfortunately, post-partum period is the most neglected period. In the developing world, while 65% of all women have some form of antenatal care, 53% get intra-natal care; only 30% get post-partum care. Women continue to need care and support after childbirth. Postpartum checkups can make all the difference for an abnormal bleeding or infection. Living away from services or being unable to afford those services prevents a woman from acquiring the knowledge needed after birth to look after herself or to receive the life-saving antibiotics and the attention she may need after delivery.

KEY FACTS

- In the sub-acute postpartum period (puerperium), 87 to 94 percent of women report at least one health problem (Glazener et al, 1995; Thompson et al, 2002).
- Long term health problems (persisting after the delayed postpartum period) are reported by 31 percent of women (Borders, 2006).
- Prevalence of Post-traumatic Stress Disorder (PTSD) following normal childbirth (excluding stillbirth or major complications) is estimated to

DOI: 10.4018/978-1-7998-4357-3.ch007

be between 2.8 and 5.6 percent at six weeks postpartum (Olde et al, 2006).

- Maternal collapse is an acute life-threatening event in which the mother falls unconscious at any stage of pregnancy or up to 6 weeks of postpartum due to cardio-respiratory or neurological compromise. The effective resuscitation determines the outcome for both the mother and the foetus.

INTRODUCTION

A puerperal disorder or postpartum disorder is a disorder which presents primarily during the puerperium or postpartum period. The postpartum period is the most critical and yet the most neglected period in the lives of both mothers and the newborns, as is described by World Health Organization (WHO). Most of the maternal and neonatal deaths occur during the postpartum period (WHO, 2014).

In the scientific literature, this term is usually abbreviated as **P*x***, where ***x*** is a number of day; "Day P_5" is read as "the fifth day after birth". There is no confusion with the medical nomenclature that uses "G P" for number and outcomes of pregnancy i.e. gravidity and parity.

A postpartum or postnatal period commences immediately after the birth of a child as the body of the mother returns to its non-pregnant state, including the levels of hormone secretion and the size of the uterus (Kansky, 2016). The first six weeks after childbirth are commonly termed as puerperium or puerperal or immediate postpartum (Romano et al, 2010).

A woman who gives birth in a hospital may leave it as soon as she is medically stable, as early as few hours of postpartum, although the average stay in a hospital for the vaginal birth is one to two days. Average postnatal stay in a hospital in case of caesarean section is three to four days (National Health Service, 2016). During this period, the mother is monitored for the bleeding, functioning of bowel and bladder as well as care of the newborn. The health of the newborn is also under surveillance (Vernon, 2007). Typically, early postnatal hospital discharge is defined as discharge of the mother and newborn from the hospital within 48 hours of delivery.

The postpartum period can be divided into three distinct phases; the initial or acute phase, which lasts 6 to 12 hours after childbirth; sub-acute postpartum period, which lasts 2 to 6 weeks and the delayed postpartum period, which can last up to six months (Romano et al, 2010).

In the sub-acute postpartum period, 87 to 94 percent of women report at least one health problem (Glazener et al, 1995; Thompson et al, 2002). Long term health problems (persisting after the delayed postpartum period) are reported by 31 percent of women (Borders, 2006).

Acute Phase

The first 6 to 12 hours after childbirth is the initial or acute phase of the postpartum period (Romano et al, 2010). During this time, the mother is typically monitored by nurses or midwives as complications can usually arise during this period.

Immediately after delivery of the placenta, the uterus begins to return to its nonpregnant size and condition, a process termed uterine involution. Contraction of the interlacing myometrial muscle bundles constricts the intra-myometrial vessels and impedes blood flow, which is the major mechanism preventing hemorrhage at the placental site. Myometrial retraction (brachystasis) is a unique characteristic of the uterine muscle that enables it to maintain its shortened length following successive contractions. In addition, large vessels at the placental site thrombose, which is a secondary hemostatic mechanism for preventing blood loss. Inadequate myometrial contraction will result in atony (i.e. a soft, boggy uterus), which is the most common cause of early postpartum hemorrhage (Berens, 2019).

The pospartum bleeding is the biggest risk to health in the acute postpartum phase. The area to which the placenta was attached to the uterine wall bleeds after delivery and the uterus must contract to prevent the loss of blood. After contraction occurs, the uterus fundus or its top may be palpated at the navel level as a firm mass. It is important for the uterus to remain firm and the frequent evaluations of both the fundus and the amount of bleeding are made by the nurse or a midwife. Uterine massage is usually done to help the uterus contract (Mayo Clinic Staff, 2015).

After delivery, stitching is done if the mother had an episiotomy or tearing at vaginal opening. An episiotomy was at one time a routine. However, current researches indicate a surgical incision to be more extensive than a natural tear. It is likely to cause later sexual incontinence and pain than a natural tear. Comfort measures may be recommended by a health care practitioner to help relieve perineal pain (Mayo Clinic staff, 2015).

Though postpartum women often complain mainly of the perineal pain yet the postpartum women themselves, their families and health care professionals tend to under-value perineal pain as during this period, the newborn care becomes a top priority, while the needs of the postpartum women go to the background. Identifying and valuing morbidities derived from normal delivery, particularly the presence of pain, is the priority for health care professionals who attend women in the puerperal period. It is considered important to identify the spontaneous perineal pain and the methods used for relieving it so as to minimize the pain, thereby offering women the opportunity to experience motherhood in a positive and pleasant way. The objective of this study was to identify the prevalence and intensity of postpartum perineal pain while in hospital and to verify the therapeutic measures used for relieving it (Francisco et al, 2011).

Within about 10 seconds of delivery, the infant takes its first breath and the caregiver places the baby on the mother's chest. The holding of an infant with ventral skin-to-skin contact, typically in an upright position with the swaddled infant on the mother's chest, is commonly referred to as kangaroo care (KC), because of its marsupial care simulation. It is recommended that kangaroo care should be used as the standard of care in the delivery of quality health care for all infants, regardless of geographical location or economic status, as it is a feasible, natural and cost-effective intervention. Numerous advantages of its use have been reported in terms of mortality, physiological (thermoregulation, cardiorespiratory stability), behavioral (sleep, length of breastfeeding and degree of exclusivity) domains as an effective therapy for relieving procedural pain as well as for improving neurodevelopment of an infant (Campbell-Yeo, 2015). The Apgar scale is used to evaluate the condition of infant. The score is calculated through evaluation on five criteria of the newborn baby which has been summarized with the use of selected words to form a backronym (**A**ppearance, **P**ulse, **G**rimace, **A**ctivity and **R**espiration).

Till recently, after birth, newborn babies were routinely taken away from their mothers. Starting around the year 2000, however, health authorities started recommending that early skin-to-skin contact by placing the naked newborn baby on the mother's chest is beneficial both the mother and an infant. Early skin-to-skin contact, also known as **kangaroo care**, is endorsed by all major health organizations responsible for the wellbeing of infants as of year 2014. Therefore, in order to help establish emotional bonding and successful breastfeeding, the caregiver immediately assesses the mother and infant as the infant is lying on the chest of the mother and removes the infant for further evaluation only after the baby had its first breastfeed. The World Health Organization (WHO) also encourages skin-to-skin contact to help regulate the body temperature of the baby for the initial 24 hours after birth (Phillips, 2014).

Sub-Acute Postpartum Period

The sub-acute postpartum starts after the acute postpartum period concludes and can last for 2 to 6 weeks (Romano et al, 2010). In the sub-acute postpartum period, 87 to 94 percent of women report at least one health problem (Glazener et al, 1995; Thompson et al, 2002).

Physical Recovery in the Sub-Acute Postpartum Period

The risk of Deep Vein Thrombosis (DVT) is relatively high in the first few days after childbirth because during pregnancy, the hyper-coagulability increases and reaches its peak in the postpartum period, especially for women with reduced mobility cäsarean section (Fiengo et al, 2013). In order to reduce the risk of Deep Vein Thrombosis (DVT), anti-coagulants may be recommended or physical methods such as compression are commonly used.

Within about three weeks, the increased vascularity and edema in the vagina of woman gradually diminishes. Gradually, the cervix narrows and lengthens over a couple of weeks. Postpartum infections may lead to sepsis and may cause death, if left untreated (WHO, 2013).

About 33 percent of all women experience urinary incontinence during postpartum period. It is estimated that women who deliver vaginally are about twice as likely to have urinary incontinence as compared to women who undergo cesarean-section (Thom and Rortveit, 2010). Urinary incontinence during this period increases the risk of long-term incontinence (Romano et al, 2010).

Gradually, Uterine discharge, called lochia, slowly reduces, turning from bright red to brownish, to yellow and almost ending at about five or six weeks. Women are recommended to wear adult diapers or wedges, disposable maternity briefs, maternity pads or towels or sanitary napkins during this period. It has been contraindicated to use the tampons or menstrual cups as these may invite bacteria and pose the risk of infection (NHS Choices, 2017). An increase in lochia may indicate a delayed postpartum hemorrhage between 7 to14 days of postpartum (Kansky, 2016). Hemorrhoids and constipation usually occur during this period and stool softeners are given in routine for relief (Baby Center, 2018).

Infant Caring in the Sub-Acute Period

At 2 to 4 days postpartum, a woman's milk will generally come in. Historically, women who did not breastfeed were administered drugs to suppress lactation though this is no longer indicated medically. During this period, breastfeeding difficulties may arise. As newborns need to be fed every two hours even during the night, waking at night with the newborn is normal, thus maternal sleep is often disturbed (McGuire 2013). At this time, the lactation consultant and health visitor can be of help.

Psychological Disorders

During the sub-acute postpartum period, psychological disorders may emerge. Among these psychological disorders are postpartum depression, post-traumatic stress disorder (PTSD) and in rare cases, puerperal psychosis (Dobson and Sales, 2000). Postpartum mental illness can affect both mothers and fathers and is not uncommon (Canadian Mental Health Association, 2014). Early detection and adequate treatment is required.

Approximately 25 to 85 percent women experience the "blues" for a few days during postpartum period. About 7 to 17 percent may experience clinical depression, especially those having a higher risk with a clinical history of depression. Prevalence of Post-Traumatic Stress Disorder (PTSD) following normal childbirth (excluding stillbirth or major complications) is estimated to be between 2.8 and 5.6 percent at six weeks postpartum (Olde et al, 2006).

Delayed Postpartum Period

The delayed postpartum period starts after the sub-acute postpartum period and lasts up to six months (Romano et al, 2010). During this time, muscles and connective tissues of women return to a state of pre-pregnancy. During this period, recovery from the complications of childbirth, such as urinary and fecal incontinence, painful sexual activity and the prolapse of pelvis are usually very gradual and may not resolve in some cases (Romano et al, 2010). Symptoms of Post-traumatic Stress Disorder (PTSD) often subside during this period, dropping from 2.8 and 5.6 percent at six weeks postpartum to 1.5 percent at six months postpartum (Olde et al, 2006; Alder et al, 2006).

After nearly three months of giving birth which is typically in between two and five months, estrogen hormone level declines and larger hair loss is common, especially in the temple area (postpartum alopecia). Generally, hair grows again normally and is, thus, not recommended for treatment (Schiff, 1963; Eastham, 2001). During this period, other conditions that may develop include thyroiditis postpartum. Infant sleep progressively increases during the night and maternal sleep also improves during this period (McGuire, 2013). It is reported that 31 per cent of women experience long-term health problems usually persisting after the delayed postpartum period (Borders, 2006).

In a study carried out by Soha et al (2006), out of cohort of 9,386 deliveries, 102 patients (almost 1%) required hospital readmission because of postnatal complications during the study period from January 2005 to June 2006. Mean maternal age was reported to be 32 years (ranging 17 to 36 years) and 65 (64%) were found to be primigravidas. Results of the study revealed that spontaneous vaginal delivery occurred in 68 (66%), vacuum in 15 (14.7%), forceps in 3 (3%) and cesarean delivery in 14 (13%) [11(10%) emergency caesarean section; 3 (3%) elective caesarean section] of the total number. Post-delivery, the mean time of admission was found to be 6 days (ranging 3 to 15 days) and mean duration of admission was 3.5 days (ranging 2 to 9 days). Maternal postnatal readmission is rare (1%) with the vast majority of cases (85%) admitted due to infectious reasons in the contemporary obstetric practice. Strategies should, therefore, focus on prevention using appropriate prophylaxis of antibiotic as well as timely diagnosis so as to minimize postnatal readmission through improved vigilance by healthcare providers.

Post-Partum Hemorrhage (PPH)

Unfortunately, Post-Partum Hemorrhage is a risky endeavor due to the complexities of human pregnancy and childbirth. Severe bleeding following delivery, also known as Post-Partum Hemorrhage (PPH), is one of the most prevalent causes of maternal mortality. Worldwide, Post-Partum Hemorrhage (PPH) accounts for nearly 27 per cent of maternal deaths or more than 75,000 annual deaths. As with pregnancy-related deaths on the whole, more than 99 percent of women dying due to Post-Partum Hemorrhage (PPH) live in developing countries (PATH, 2011).

Post-Partum Hemorrhage (PPH) is defined as loss of more than 500 milliliters of blood (constituting about 10 percent of total blood volume in a person) within 24 hours of delivery. Post-Partum Hemorrhage (PPH) may be caused by anemia, damage to the birth canal, failure of the uterus to contract properly after delivery or failure to deliver a portion of the placenta, thus preventing the related maternal blood vessels in the uterus from contracting to their normal sizes (PATH, 2011).

Ironically, most of the Post-Partum Hemorrhage (PPH) deaths can be prevented by proper medical care before, during and after a child's birth. For example, the routine provision of iron and folate dietary supplements to all pregnant women can prevent anemia. Additionally, World Health Organization established the recommended practices during delivery that will help in preventing Post-Partum Hemorrhage (PPH). A set of treatments, called The Third Stage of Labor Active Management (AMTSL), involves injecting a hormone oxytocin after the delivery of baby. This hormone facilitates contraction of the uterus, helps to close the blood vessels and prevents the excessive bleeding. Studies have proved that the incidence of Post-Partum Hemorrhage (PPH) can be decreased by 62 percent by implementation of AMTSL. However, many women in the developing countries do not adhere to these practices, in the absence of adequate education about proper medical care or an access to the skilled attendants during delivery, thereby making them prone to Post-Partum Hemorrhage (PATH, 2011).

Pregnancy Induced Hypertension

The second most common cause of maternal death after severe bleeding, called Post-Partum Hemorrhage (PPH), is high blood pressure (hypertension) induced by pregnancy. Pregnancy-induced hypertension accounts for nearly 14 percent of maternal mortality or about 40,000 women dying in a year. World Health Organization has reported that more than 99 percent of deaths caused by Post-Partum Hemorrhage (PPH) occur in developing countries (WHO, 2014).

Hypertensive disorders of pregnancy are a heterogenous type of conditions that include chronic hypertension, gestational hypertension, preeclampsia and preeclampsia superimposed on chronic hypertension. Hypertensive disorders in pregnancy result in a substantial health burden, accounting for a large proportion of maternal and neonatal morbidity and mortality. In the United States, such disorders contribute a significant proportion of perinatal morbidity and mortality among 10 percent of maternal deaths. There is a rising concern of optimizing management of these disorders under the given conditions of substantial health burden of hypertensive disorders during pregnancy (Sutton, Harper and Tita, 2018).

A typically dangerous type of hypertension for the mother and the foetus is preeclampsia-induced hypertension, a disorder which is characterized by high blood pressure after 20 week of gestation, thus leading to high protein levels in the urine due to kidney problems. In severe cases, preeclampsia-induced hypertension might cause a permanent damage to the organs of a mother, especially brain and liver. It may also result in seizures, a condition called eclampsia and death.

Preeclampsia

Preeclampsia may impair the placental functions, thereby causing the birth of underweight or premature infants. Preeclampsia leads to additional premature births because the delivery of the foetus is unfortunately the only 'cure' for this condition. Therefore, under severe conditions, doctors are compelled to deliver a foetus dangerously early in order to save both the mother and the fetus ' lives (Medline Plus Medical Encyclopedia, 2012).

While preeclampsia is hard to diagnose with its causes being poorly understood, its dangers may be reduced through adequate medical assistance. Prenatal screening, for example, can diagnose high blood pressure in mothers early in pregnancy so that her condition is regularly monitored and by avoiding those activities which further raise her blood pressure. Furthermore, a drug called magnesium sulfate can prevent seizure development in women with preeclampsia and reduce their mortality risk by more than 50 percent (Preeclampsia Foundation, 2013). Unfortunately, the lack of information, inadequate training for healthcare workers and limited availability of the drug magnesium sulfate are the reasons for its restricted use in developing countries (Caucus on New and Underused Reproductive Health Technologies, 2012).

Strategies to prevent preeclampsia include the identification of high risk patients and initiation of low dose of aspirin in early gestation. Women with preterm preeclampsia with severe features can be expectantly managed to decrease the risks of prematurity.

Maternal Cardiac Disease

Due to lifestyle changes i.e. late age of conception and the overall maternal health status, including obesity, diabetes and smoking, pre-existing congenital heart disease, cardiac disease is increasingly common among women during pregnancy. A multidisciplinary approach is required to evaluate the complications and provide antenatal and peripartum care in cases of known maternal cardiac disease. However, most of the deaths secondary to cardiac disease take place among women who had no previous history of cardiac diseases.

During Pregnancy, the risk of myocardial infarction is raised three- to four-fold as compared to non-pregnant population. Moreover, the risk is significantly higher among women above 36 years of age or with black ethnicity. In addition, there is a greater risk of coronary artery or aortic dissection in pregnancy. It is important to remember that pregnant patients with cardiac disease frequently present with atypical symptoms.

Maternal Collapse

Maternal collapse is an acute life-threatening condition in which the mother gets unconscious at any stage of pregnancy or up to 6 weeks of postpartum due to cardio-respiratory or neurological compromise. This may prove fatal for the mother and the foetus and the effective resuscitation may help in recovery.

Patients are most likely to survive if attended by health care providers who are professionally trained and skilled in the basic and advanced life-support techniques. Its successful outcome depends upon the mechanical and physiological changes during pregnancy and thus should be taken into consideration.

In a hospital setting, maternal collapse and sudden cardiac arrest are often associated with peripartum events after delivery. Thus, health care providers working on the delivery suite should be professionally trained in the advanced life-support techniques. In case of any such emergency, the resuscitation equipment should be instantly available.

Though the incidence of maternal collapse and severe maternal morbidity is not known yet the estimates indicate that the incidence of maternal cardiac arrest is 1 in 30, 000 deliveries (Cluver et al, 2013). Despite a young age group, survival rates are poor.

Causes for Maternal Collapse

While some underlying causes of maternal collapse cannot be prevented, it is important to note that due to deterioration of underlying critical disease, there is frequent maternal cardiac arrest. Therefore, it is crucial to maintain a maternal early-warning chart for observing all pregnant women in a hospital setting so as to diagnose the critical illness as soon as possible.

Haemorrhage

Hemorrhage remains the leading cause of maternal mortality worldwide. It is also the major cause of maternal collapse in a delivery unit. Multiple pregnancy, high parity, placenta praevia, uterine fibroids and multiple previous caesarean sections, prolonged labor, motherly clotting disorders and preeclampsia are the various predisposing factors. As a young pregnant woman may lose a significant amount of blood without any haemo-dynamic disturbance, it is very important to take care of all these risk factors. Thus, a high suspicion index can be life-saving. In case the haemo-dynamic changes become apparent, it is indicated that one- third of her circulating blood volume has already been lost by the mother.

Venous Thromboembolism

Thromboembolism is a significant contributor and the leading cause of maternal morbidity and mortality worldwide. Venous Thromboembolism (VTE) comprises of deep vein thrombosis (DVT), pulmonary thromboembolism (PE) along with other forms of mesenteric vein thrombosis and intracranial venous thrombosis which are rarer. As compared to the non-pregnant population, its overall incidence is 2 to 4 times higher among pregnant women. Throughout pregnancy, its risk is raised but it is maximum during the postpartum period. The incidence of Venous Thromboembolism (VTE) varies between 1 to 2 per 1000 to 80 percent for Deep Vein Thrombosis (DVT's) in the antepartum period and 20 to 25 percent for pulmonary thromboembolism (PE). On the contrary, the incidence of pulmonary thromboembolism (PE) is much greater during postpartum period, with 40 to 60 percent of all PE's taking place after delivery (Kolettis and Craigo, 2018).

Those women, who are at highest risk of thrombo-embolism should be identified and their pregnancies should be properly managed by providing them an appropriate thrombo-prophylaxis. This is especially required to reduce this life-threatening condition. Women, who at the highest risk are one with thrombophilias, who have a personal or family history of venous thromboembolism and women undergoing a cesarean delivery (Kolettis and Craigo, 2018).

A careful risk assessment for thrombotic complications should be performed in all pregnant women. Multiple risk factors may necessitate the thrombo-prophylactic treatment during pregnancy as well as postpartum. It should always be remembered that Deep Vein Thrombosis (DVT) of the pelvic venous system is often asymptomatic until pulmonary embolism develops.

As a part of standard obstetric practice, thrombo-prophylaxis should be given to patients who are at highest risk of venous thromboembolism. Necessary measures should be undertaken based on the individual risk factors so as to mitigate the risk of venous thromboembolism after cesarean delivery, which include early ambulation and mechanical or pharmacologic thrombo-prophylaxis.

Although there are variations in the current international guidelines on thrombo-prophylaxis but all strategies depend upon the identification of various risk factors and thrombo-prophylaxis should be given to the highest risk pregnant women. Moreover, the physicians need to think critically about the individual risk factors throughout the pregnancy and the postpartum period so as to frame the necessary guidelines (Kolettis and Craigo, 2018).

Amniotic Fluid Embolism (AFE)

An estimated incidence of Amniotic Fluid Embolism (AFE) of 2.0 cases per 1, 00, 000 maternities has been reported through an analysis of data collected over a period of 4 years by UKOSS (Knight, 2010). Since this event cannot be prevented, its outcome depends upon the speed of diagnosis. Moreover, there is no diagnostic test for identification of Amniotic Fluid Embolism (AFE). Thus, the clinical signs lead to a high degree of suspicion.

Clinical signs of Amniotic Fluid Embolism (AFE) are respiratory distress, followed by cardiovascular collapse with cardio-genic shock, which may occur frequently in combination with haemorrhage caused by coagulopathy. Amniotic Fluid Embolism (AFE) can also result in the collapse of the foetus which may be of unknown origin and it usually precedes maternal collapse. In all such cases, there is lack of any other significant medical condition or explanation for the rapid deterioration of this condition.

Peri-Mortem Caesarean Section

The utero-placental unit sequesters blood and hinders effective Cardio Pulmonary Resuscitation (CPR). Case reports support the positive effect of evacuating the uterus on maternal outcome during CPR during late stage of pregnancy i.e. after 20 weeks of gestation. However, there is negative correlation between survival and the time between maternal arrest and the delivery. An emergency caesarean delivery within 4 minutes of maternal collapse is recommended, as per the current recommendations if there is no response to resuscitation efforts which is to be completed within 5 minutes.

In an attempt to critically examine the causes and potential prevention of maternal death in the United States since the year 2000, Clark et al (2006) found that out of 1,239,385 deliveries (6.3/100,000 births), 78 maternal deaths occurred. The rate of maternal mortality for women undergoing cesarean delivery was 13.2/100,000 cesarean sections and for vaginal deliveries, the rate of maternal mortality was 1.5/100,000 vaginal births. Amniotic fluid embolism (15%), complications of preeclampsia (15%), pulmonary thromboembolism (13%), cardiac disease (11%), obstetric hemorrhage (9%), non-OB infection (8%), and accident / suicide (7%) were found to be the leading causes of death. Death was caused by the complications of the operation itself rather than by the indication for the cesarean section in only 4 cases of cesarean sections. All of these cases have been potentially deemed to be preventable. In 9 additional cases of pulmonary thrombo-embolism, cesarean section could have contributed to mortality. Only one fatal pulmonary embolism was reported among women who delivered vaginally. In 10 cases, 13% of deaths occurred due to an error on the part of medical provider. In another 10 cases, 13% of deaths were caused by the patient's action or that of another non-medical provider.

In this particular study, various causes of maternal deaths have also been reported by Clark et al (2006). With more appropriate medical care, seventeen deaths (18%) were adjudged for being preventable. These maternal deaths fall under the categories of postpartum hemorrhage (8), preeclampsia (5), medication error (3) and infection (1). The distribution of these preventable maternal deaths based on ethnicity were reported to be white 9 (53%), African American 5 (29%) and Hispanic 3 (18%) (Clark et al, 2006).

Besides, maternal deaths in relation to mode of delivery have also been reported by Clark et al (2006). Cesarean delivery directly accounted for four deaths out of which, death was caused by hemorrhage from bleeding vessels injured during surgery in 3 cases (all primary cesareans). In remaining one case of repeated cesarean delivery, death during the operation occurred due to sepsis which was secondary to surgical injury to the bowel. Besides, one case of uterine inversion-related hemorrhagic death and one case of rupture of an unrecognized berry aneurism during labour, resulted in two deaths related to vaginal delivery. On the contrary, among 12 preeclampsia related deaths, 3 deaths occurred due to hemorrhage and one death due to sepsis (a total of 17 percent of all deaths). All these deaths were potentially preventable if a cesarean delivery had been performed or an earlier cesarean delivery could have been undertaken. A peri-mortem operative procedure was used after maternal cardiac arrest in 20 out of 58 maternal deaths (35 percent) which were associated with cesarean delivery. None of these deaths could be attributed to the cesarean delivery itself. Nine patients in all died from pulmonary thromboembolism, out of which 6 died following primary cesarean delivery, one died after repeat cesarean delivery and 2 died following vaginal birth. Among these patients, no one had received prophylaxis of the peripartum thromboembolism either in the form of fractional or non-fractional heparin or pneumatic compression devices. Thus, excess maternal deaths due to pulmonary embolism in women who underwent cesarean delivery were attributed causally to the cesarean delivery among these women (Clark et al, 2006).

Currently, most of the maternal deaths cannot be prevented. Though cesarean section is linked with a higher mortality rate as compared to the vaginal delivery, it is not only commonly causative. However, deaths causally linked to cesarean section are all potentially preventable. Under the given conditions of diverse causes of maternal mortality, significant decline in the maternal mortality rate in the United States can only be achieved through better understanding of the nature and the prevention of preeclampsia and amniotic fluid embolism and/or universal thrombo-prophylaxis for all women who undergo cesarean section (Clark et al, 2006).

CONCLUSION

The decision to use contraception is one of the most important choices a woman or couple can make. Even though a couple decides to have a child as soon as possible after marriage, the use of contraception thereafter for the "spacing" of children is a judicious decision. Evidence reveals that optimal spacing between two children should be at least three to four years. Family planning enables parents to ensure the child with the best possible chance for its nourishment and nurturing before the birth of another child.

Spacing is also crucial for the health of the child and the mother as well as for the financial wellbeing and harmony of the family as a unit. At the same time, the use of contraception to limit the size of the family that the couple can truly afford and provide for, is also a judicious decision. Moreover, the use of contraception also contributes to a more satisfying sexual relationship for many couples by reducing or eliminating the fear of accidental or unwanted pregnancies.

It is, thus, crucial for the health and well-being of children, families and the communities that family planning information and services are made available to help them all know about and effectively make use of various method of contraception for planning their families.

REFERENCES

Alder, J., Stadlmayr, W., Tschudin, S., & Bitzer, J. (2006). Post-traumatic symptoms after childbirth: What should we offer? *Journal of Psychosomatic Obstetrics and Gynaecology*, *27*(2), 107–112. doi:10.1080/01674820600714632 PMID:16808085

Baby Center. (2018). *Postpartum Hemmorhoids*. Author.

Berens, P. (2019). *Overview of the postpartum period: Physiology, complications, and maternal care.* Academic Press.

Borders, N. (2006). After the afterbirth: A critical review of postpartum health relative tomethod of delivery. *Journal of Midwifery & Women's Health*, *51*(4), 242–248. doi:10.1016/j.jmwh.2005.10.014 PMID:16814217

Campbell-Yeo, M. L., Disher, T. C., Benoit, B. L., & Johnston, C. C. (2015). Understanding kangaroo care and its benefits to preterm infants. *Pediatric Health, Medicine and Therapeutics*, *6*, 15–32. doi:10.2147/PHMT.S51869 PMID:29388613

Canadian Mental Health Association. (2014). *Postpartum Depression*. Author.

Caucus on New and Underused Reproductive Health Technologies. (2012). *Magnesium Sulfate*. https://www.path.org/publications/files/RHSC_ms_br.pdf

Clark, S., Dildy, G., Belfort, M., Meyers, J., Herbst, M., Frye, D. & Hankins, G. (2006). Reducing Maternal Mortality in the 21st Century. *Obstetrics and Gynecology.*

Cluver, C., Novikova, N., Hofmeyr, G. J., & Hall, D. R. (2013). Maternal position during Caesarean section for preventing maternal and neonatal complications. *Cochrane Database of Systematic Reviews, 3*, CD007623. doi:10.1002/14651858.CD007623.pub3 PMID:23543552

Dobson, V., & Sales, B. (2000). The Science of Infanticide and Mental Illness. *Psychology, Public Policy, and Law, 6*(4), 1098–1112. doi:10.1037/1076-8971.6.4.1098

Eastham, J. H. (2001). Postpartum Alopecia. *The Annals of Pharmacotherapy, 35*, 255– 258. doi:10.1345/1542-6270(2001)035<0255:pa>2.0.co;2

Fiengo, L., Bucci, F., Patrizi, G., Giannotti, D., & Redler, A. (2013). Postpartum deep vein thrombosis and pulmonary embolism in twin pregnancy: An undertaking of clinical symptoms leading to massive complications. *Thrombosis Journal, 11*(1), 4. doi:10.1186/1477-9560-11-4 PMID:23433174

Glazener, C. M., Abdalla, M., Stroud, P., Naji, S., Templeton, A., & Russell, I. T. (1995). Postnatal maternal morbidity: Extent, causes, prevention and treatment. *British Journal of Obstetrics and Gynaecology, 102*(4), 282–287. doi:10.1111/j.1471-0528.1995.tb09132.x PMID:7612509

Kansky, C. (2016). *Normal and Abnormal Puerperium: Overview, Routine Postpartum Care, Hemorrhage. Obstetrics and Gynaecology*. Medscape.

Knight, M. (2010). Amniotic Fluid Embolism in the U. K. *Obstetrician & Gynaecologist, 115*, 910–917. doi:10.1097/AOG.0b013e3181d9f629

Kolettis, D., & Craigo, S. (2018). Thromophylaxis in Pregnancy. *Obstretrics and Gynecology Clinics, 45*(2), 389–402. PMID:29747737

Mathai, M. (1999). National Medical Journal of india, 1,12, 251.

Mayo Clinic Staff. (2015). *Labor and delivery, postpartum care*. Mayo Clinic.

McGuire, E. (2013). Maternal and infant sleep postpartum. *Breastfeeding Review, 21*(2), 38–41. PMID:23957180

MedlinePlus Medical Encyclopedia. (2012). *Preeclampsia*. https://www.nlm.nih.gov/medlineplus/ency/article/000898.htm

Mukherji, J., Ganguly, R. P., Saha, S. K., Samir, C., & Ghosh, R. (2002). Postpartum Care- A Neglected Tragedy. *Journal of Obstetrics and Gynaecology of India, 52*(4), 40–43.

NHS. (2016). Recovering from a caesarean section. *Choices.*

NHS Choices (2017). How soon can I use tampons after giving birth? *N.H.S. Choices.*

Olde, E., Vander Hart, O., Kleber, R. & Van Son, M. (2006). Posttraumatic stress following childbirth: A review. *Clinical Psychology Review*, *26*(1), 1–16. doi:10.1016/j.cpr.2005.07.002

Oliveira, Oliveira Santos, & da Silva. (2011). Evaluation and treatment of perineal pain in vaginal postpartum. *Acta Paulista de Enfermagem*, *24*(1); Advance online publication. doi:10.1590/S0103-21002011000100014

Phillips, R. (2014). *Uninterrupted Skin-to-Skin Contact Immediately After Birth*. Medscape.

Preeclampsia Foundation. (2013). *FAQs*. https://www.preeclampsia.org/health-information/faqs

Program for Appropriate Technology in Health (PATH). (2011). *Postpartum Hemorrhage*. http://www.pphprevention.org/pph.php

Renate, W. (2012). Principles of resuscitation for maternal collapse. In *Obstetric and Intrapartum Emergencies: A Practical Guide to Management*. Cambridge University Press.

Romano, M., Cacciatore, A., Giordano, R., & La Rosa, B. (2010). Postpartum period: Three distinct but continuous phases. *Journal of Prenatal Medicine*, *4*(2), 22–25. PMID:22439056

Schiff, B. L. (1963). Study of Postpartum Alopecia. *Archives of Dermatology*, *87*(5), 609. doi:10.1001/archderm.1963.01590170067011

Soha, S., Fionnuala, M., Breathnach, M. G., Fergal, D., & Malone. (2006). Maternal readmission and postnatal morbidity in contemporary obstetric practice. *The American Journal of Obstetrics and Gynecology.*

Sutton, A. L. M., Harper, L. M., & Tita, A. T. N. (2018). Hypertensive Disorders in Pregnancy. *Obstetrics and Gynecology Clinics*, *45*(2), 333–347. PMID:29747734

Thom, D. H., & Rortveit, G. (2010). Prevalence of postpartum urinary incontinence: A systematic review. *Acta Obstetricia et Gynecologica Scandinavica*, *89*(12), 1511–1522. doi:10.3109/00016349.2010.526188 PMID:21050146

Thompson, J. F., Roberts, C. L., Currie, M., & Ellwood, D. A. (2002). Prevalence and persistence of health problems after childbirth: Associations with parity and method of birth. *Birth (Berkeley, Calif.)*, *29*(2), 83–94. doi:10.1046/j.1523-536X.2002.00167.x PMID:12051189

Vernon, D. (2007). *With women, midwives experiences: from shift-work to continuity of care*. Australian College of Midwives.

World Health Organization. (2013). *WHO recommendations on postnatal care of the mother and newborn*. World Health Organization.

World Health Organization. (2014). *WHO recommendations on postnatal care of the mother and newborn*. WHO.

World Health Organization. (2014). *Maternal Mortality Fact Sheet.* https://www.who.int/mediacentre/factsheets/fs348/en/www.aboutkidshealth.ca

Chapter 8
Management of High-Risk Pregnancies

ABSTRACT

Rarely does a pregnancy happen without any complication. The majority of these problems are minor and due to normal anatomical and physiological changes occurring during pregnancy. However, some are more serious and require medical attention. Certain conditions that are specific to pregnancy and occur during pregnancy classify it as a high-risk pregnancy. A high-risk pregnancy is closely monitored with antenatal check-ups and possibly an additional care. In labour, certain obstetric complications require an immediate intervention. A high-quality antenatal care means that potentially serious conditions are usually successfully managed, both during pregnancy and in labour. Post-delivery problems, either to baby or to mother, may also need medical attention with careful follow-up and sometimes referral. Thus, providing good antenatal care, finding appropriate ways of preventing, and dealing with consequences of unwanted pregnancies and improving the way society looks after pregnant women are the three most important ways to reduce maternal mortality in high risk pregnancies.

KEY FACTS

- Nevertheless, maternal mortality ratios, ranging from less than five maternal deaths per 100 000 live-births in high-income countries to more than 500 per 100 000 live births in several countries in Sub-

DOI: 10.4018/978-1-7998-4357-3.ch008

saharan Africa, remain among the least equitable of all health indicators, (WHO, UNICEF, UNFPA, World Bank, 2010).

- In the African Region, the maternal mortality ratio at an average of 940 per 100,000 live births, is the highest in the world (WHO, 2000).
- The estimated number of women, who die each year from causes related to pregnancy or childbirth, has dropped substantially from 543, 000 deaths in the year 1990 to about 287, 000 in the year 2010 (WHO, UNICEF, 2013; WHO, UNICEF, UNFPA, World Bank, 2010).
- Sadly, most countries are expected not to achieve the maternal mortality target set for the Millennium Development Goals (WHO, UNICEF, 2013).

INTRODUCTION

In many parts of the world, an early marriage is still a norm. Generally, early marriage results in early motherhood. However, in many developing countries, at least 20 per cent of women give birth to their first child before the age of 18 years while in some other countries, about half of all women give birth to their first child before the age of 18 years. The parents, in-laws and society's expectations are to give birth to a child as soon as possible after marriage. Many young women are under pressure to carry sons. This typically leads to pregnancies being spaced too close together, in addition to occurring too soon in the life of the young mother.

Women, who marry or enter union at a young age, are likely to have their partners who are much older in age than they are; which is sometimes as old as 15 years older in some countries. This difference in age of the partners reduces the chance that the woman will be able to participate in decision making process about childbearing or be able to negotiate the use of the contraceptives.

Data from 21 countries with full statistics revealed that the pregnancy rate among adolescents, aged 15 to 19 years, was the maximum in the United States (57 pregnancies per 1,000 females) and minimum in Switzerland (8 pregnancies per 1,000 females). Data from some former Soviet countries with incomplete statistics revealed these rates to be higher. With the available information, these rates were highest in Mexico and Sub-saharan African countries. Hungary had the highest pregnancy rate among 10 to 14-year-old adolescents, as reported among countries with reliable evidence. The proportion of abortion-induced adolescent pregnancies ranged from Slovakia

(17 percent) to Sweden (69 percent). The proportion of pregnancies resulting in live births remained higher in countries with high rates of adolescent pregnancies. Since mid-1990's, the pregnancy rates have fallen in majority of the 16 countries where these trends could be assessed (Sedgh et al, 2015).

Reviews of earlier country-wide studies on rates of adolescent pregnancy and childbearing covered trends up to the mid-1990's. Results revealed that such events became less common in most of the countries with available evidence (Singh and Darroch, 2000; Singh, 1998). At that time, the rate of adolescent pregnancy was higher in the United States than any other developed country with available estimates, except Russia. Region-wise estimates of developing countries indicated adolescent birth rates in Sub-Saharan Africa to be particularly high (National Research Council, 2005).

Despite the recent declines in child bearing rates, rates of adolescent pregnancy remain too high in most of the countries. Research evidence on the planning status of such pregnancies and the factors which determine the ways adolescent mothers use to resolve their pregnancies could further shape the maternal and child health programs and policies.

Causes and Consequences of Teen Pregnancies

The contributing causes and consequences of adolescent pregnancies have been an area of much research, policy/ program discussion and debate. Findings of various studies suggested that adolescent pregnancies compromise on the educational prospects and economic opportunities of women (UNFPA, 2013; World Health Organization, 2014; National Research Council, 2005) and other work indicates that teen pregnancies are a marker of such conditions rather than an underlying cause of them (Coyne and D'Onofrio, 2012; Korenman and Fales, 2011). There does appear to be consensus, however, that teen pregnancies are associated with poor social and economic conditions and prospects.

As a result of pregnancy, adolescents face a greater risk of complications and death as compared to their older counterparts. In Latin America, for example, the risk of maternal mortality is four-fold greater among adolescents below 16 years of age as compared to women in their twenties (WHO, 2014). Anemia, malaria, HIV and other STIs, postpartum hemorrhage and mental disorders such as depression are various complications associated with adolescent pregnancies (WHO, 2014; Hodgkinson et al, 2010).

Pregnancy and delivery for adolescent girls who have not completed their body growth expose them to problems that are less common in adult women; 9 to 86 percent of women with obstetric fistula develop the condition as adolescents, with traumatic, often lifelong consequences (Tebeu et al, 2012). It has been well documented that low socioeconomic status, substance abuse and likelihood of receiving low and/or inadequate prenatal care are closely associated with adolescent pregnancies and poor outcomes for the offspring of adolescent mothers. These poor outcomes include higher rates of preterm birth, low birth weight and asphyxia and perinatal and neonatal mortality for the offsprings (Chen et al, 2007; WHO, 2014; Lopez et al, 2012).

Causes of Maternal Mortality

Maternal mortality has been defined as death of a woman during pregnancy or within 42 days of the termination of pregnancy. Various major direct causes of maternal mortality are anaemia, eclampsia, hemorrhage, unsafe abortion, obstructed labour and puerperal infections. HIV/AIDS, malaria, viral hepatitis (especially hepatitis E virus), heart diseases, pulmonary tuberculosis, diarrhoeal diseases like dysentery, typhoid, cholera and amoebiasis, tetanus, sickle cell disease etc are the major indirect causes. Besides, various traditional practices which are harmful may contribute significantly to maternal mortality and morbidity in certain cultures. Some of complications of pregnancy resulting in chronic conditions include chronic pelvic inflammatory disease, infertility, ectopic pregnancy and obstetric fistula.

Moreover, in some countries, HIV/AIDs have increasingly been contributing to maternal mortality. Opportunistic infections are also common. With increased frequencies of abortions, ectopic pregnancies and other complications of pregnancy, the perinatal outcome is also poor.

During pregnancy, malaria is also more dangerous than outside pregnancy. In certain highly endemic areas, maternal mortality due to malaria results mainly from the most important indirect effect of the condition that is severe anaemia. In areas of unstable malaria, maternal mortality occurs from its direct effects, especially cerebral malaria with coma. In both areas, however, the most common risk to the foetus is low birth weight of the newborn.

Maternal Mortality by Age: Who is Most at Risk?

In a study published in the Journal *The Lancet Global Health*, Andrea Nove and colleagues (Nove et al, 2014) report the results of an analysis of data from 144 countries, which together account for 93 percent of the world's annual births (Nove et al, 2014). Such a voluminous and diverse data allowed for the analysis of age-specific national-wise estimates of maternal mortality at a scale that was not possible earlier.

Some important findings are revealed through this research. **First,** the mortality risk associated with adolescent pregnancy is only about one-third higher than the mortality risk of older women, aged 20 to 24 years (260 [uncertainty 100–410] vs. 190 [uncertainty 120–260] maternal deaths per 100 000 live births) and thus not that high as believed earlier. **Second**, older women over 35 years of age had the highest ratios of maternal mortality. Although this pattern has been previously described but no previous study has reported such a convincing data from so many countries. **Third,** age-specific maternal mortality varied significantly across countries and regions. Some countries revealed the classic J-shaped maternal mortality ratio by age while others revealed the lowest maternal mortality ratio of any age group. This group of countries is the countries with very high maternal mortality ratios in Sub-saharan Africa (e.g., Central African Republic, Democratic Republic of Congo and Zambia). **Fourth,** it does not appear that the data source, i.e. vital registration or censuses and surveys, affect the overall conclusions. **Finally,** most estimates of uncertainty for the 15 to 19 years adolescents overlap with those for older mothers, aged 20 to 24 years (Nove et al, 2014).

Results of previous studies on maternal mortality have shown that the association between maternal age and several adverse perinatal outcomes is importantly confounded by socio-economic status. However, the descriptive study of Nove and colleagues' analysis did not take this into account. This confounding will lead to increased risks for the young mothers, who are poorer and less educated than their older counterparts in all types of settings. For older mothers in many countries, the confounding might mask even stronger associations where older mothers tend to be better off (Lawlor et al, 2011).

Parity also plays an important role as both nulliparous and high-parity women are generally at an increased risk of adverse maternal outcomes (Nortman, 1974). Whether all adolescents have a similar mortality risk issue has also been raised by the findings of Nove and colleagues'.

Maternal mortality ratio analysis has traditionally treated adolescents as a single age group, i.e. between the ages of 15 and 19 years but this approach may mask significant differences in terms of biological maturity as well as social conditions. Such a wide age group comprises of both very young adolescent mothers, for whom childbearing has a high social and biological risk as well as those in the ages of 18 and 19 years who may have their reproductive status in their primary biological — though not social — status (Nortman, 1974). Consequently, the risk to the age group of 15 to 19 years old is affected by the proportions of young or old adolescent mothers within this group.

Evaluation and Management of High-Risk Pregnancies

Maternal mortality plagues much of the world. The year 2015 saw 303,000 maternal deaths, representing a global maternal mortality ratio of 216 maternal deaths per 100,000 live births. Maternal mortality ratio had been declining in the United States until the year 1987, it remained stable until the year 1999 and then it began to rise. There are racial disparities in maternal mortality rates in the United States with maternal deaths affecting a higher proportion of Black women as compared to their White counterparts. US national organizations called for a standardized review of maternal morbidity and mortality cases so as to reduce maternal mortality ratio (Ozimek and Kilparrick, 2018).

Maternal death rates in the United States have remained constant for several decades (Chang et al, 2003). This could be attributed to the stagnation in improvement of quality with regard to maternal mortality or a masking of enhanced quality caused by the demographic changes or it may be due to the appearance of newer diseases or more virulent forms of already established diseases. Alternately, given the known association of these procedures with increased rates of maternal mortality, an improvement in the overall quality of maternal care may be masked by the increasing rate of cesarean delivery (Hall and Bewley, 1999; Harper et al, 2003).

Recent advancements in medical science have enabled women with complex medical problems to choose their pregnancy and manage it successfully through a usually challenging gestation. However, there is an unprecedented increase in maternal morbidity and mortality in the United States in the early twenty-first century. This could be attributed to factors like sick patients being able to conceive or as a result of increased rate of obesity, advancing maternal age and other factors, thereby leading to increased morbidity related to pregnancy (Peterson and Hibbard, 2018).

Childbearing is highly unsafe in Sub-Saharan Africa (SSA). The huge mortality and morbidity rates among pregnant women in Sub-Saharan Africa (SSA) are the direct consequences of the serious issues in the social, cultural and economic status as well as the inadequate existing health care services available to the beneficiaries.

For the design of any intervention programmes, Identification of high-risk groups is, thus, an important requisite. For example, the mortality risk of adolescent mothers is often twice as high as for those mothers in their early 20's (UNFPA, 2012; WHO, 2011). This statistic fits well with the agenda of reducing adolescent childbearing, which is being championed as a priority by international and bilateral agencies (WHO, 2011; UNFPA, 2013).

An access to skilled healthcare during and after pregnancy as well as delivery is one of the biggest remaining disparities. Many pregnancy and labour related complications resulting in maternal mortality could be avoided or treated with the assistance of a trained health care provider like a midwife, a nurse or a doctor. Only about one-third of women in low-income countries, however, receive the recommended four antenatal checkups and only 46 percent of women get the assistance of qualified attendant while giving birth. In addition to absence of trained health care providers and adequate equipment, poor rural women also face the challenges of distance, expenditure, lack of education and cultural practices that create barriers in their care seeking during and after pregnancies (World Health Organization, 2014).

United Nations, in the year 2000, included improving maternal health as one of its eight Millennium Development Goals (MDGs) in order to address such disparities. The objective of MDG-5 was to reduce the maternal mortality rate by 75 percent from the years 1990 to 2015 through its efforts such as identifying underlying causes of high maternal mortality rates and working with local governments to increase an access to healthcare services for pregnant women (World Health Organization, 2015).

Significant progress has been made towards achieving the goals of MDG-5. Maternal mortality rate, for example, has fallen by 45 percent worldwide since the year 1990, with some Sub-Saharan nations declining maternal mortality by more than 50 percent. Despite this significant progress, MDG-5 has not been achieved till the beginning of this year and much effort is yet to be done (World Health Organization, 2015).

In such a scenario, the nation-specific estimates of pregnancy, childbirth and abortion among adolescent mothers can motivate the policy and programmatic responses to adolescent pregnancies and ensure monitoring the progress towards decreasing their incidences. Countries having low levels of adolescent pregnancy may serve as references or models to motivate others for targeted efforts to reduce these incidences. Even countries with low incidence, data on adolescent pregnancies can bring to light the remaining unmet needs for the required information and health care services to enable adolescents prevent the unintended pregnancies.

Existing Scenario

In the present scenario, 88 percent of the pregnancies undergo normal physiological course requiring only basic care while remaining 12 percent of cases are high risk pregnancies, thereby requiring an additional assistance and are case-specific. Thus, basic approach should be an assessment of all pregnant women for considering their potential to have a normal pregnancy until or unless there is no clear evidence to the contrary. Effective communication, control and early detection are the important tools that must be ensured so as to plan the best possible treatment strategies and to minimize the risks of maternal and/or foetal mortality (Coco et al, 2014).

Findings of various studies on maternal mortality need to be interpreted in the light of present trends in age at childbearing. United Nations reported a fall in adolescent fertility rates from 71 to 52 per thousand women, aged 15 to 19 years worldwide during the period of 1970's to 2000's (UN Population Division, 2009). This decline was observed in all regions, with an exception of Latin America. Substantial decreases for birth rates among women, aged 35 years and older, were also observed in Africa, Asia and Latin America but slight increases were seen in high-income countries (UN Population Division, 2009). These patterns, taken together with Nove and colleagues' findings (Nove et al, 2014) suggest that existing trends in age-specific fertility will contribute to a reduction in maternal mortality in the near future.

However, the most striking finding from Nove and colleagues' study (Nove et al, 2014) pertains to women, older than 35 years of age who are at very high risk. Based on these data, 70 maternal deaths would be prevented by delaying 1,00, 000 adolescent pregnancies up to the age of 20 to 24 years while more than 1000 deaths would be prevented if 1,00, 000 pregnancies currently occurring in women, aged 40 years or older, when the same women were in their early 20's. While late maternity in high-income and middle-income countries may be an inevitable consequence of a broadly positive improvement in the role of women in the society, many maternal deaths in low-income countries can still be prevented by enhancing an access to contraception in order to reduce unplanned, high-parity births (Alkema et al, 2013).

Thus, many more overwhelming reasons exist for adolescent girls to avoid and prevent early childbearing which include the widespread adverse social, educational and economic consequences for young mothers, irrespective of the size of the increased risk of maternal mortality for adolescents (UNFPA, 2013).

STRATEGIES FOR REDUCING MATERNAL MORTALITY (World Health Organization, 2000)

Fundamental Principles

Following conditions need to be satisfied to make childbearing safer:

- Inter-sectoral collaboration to improve the living conditions and raise the level of acceptance of modern maternity care by the population;
- Strengthening the health care system for capacity building of professional antenatal care to achieve total population coverage;
- Providing a suitable mix of interventions to salvage unbooked emergencies for the most vulnerable group having highest proportion of maternal deaths;
- Promoting conditions of socio-economic, educational, cultural, infrastructural, political and health to eliminate unbooked emergencies.

Pillars of Maternity Care

Following features of the health care system are unique to maternity care:

- Efficient antenatal care at the first facility and the community levels to ensure coverage of the total population;
- Efficient Referral system: Women with complications (including puerperal complications) to be transferred soon to second level facilities (district hospitals or their equivalents) for referral services;
- Efficient transport is a crucial element;
- Specific guidelines to be framed to assess the quality of antenatal care and action taken for improvement.

Strengthening Community Participation

Community participation to be strengthened by:

- Identifying the strengths and weaknesses of the community set-up through standardized methods like conducting interviews, observation schedules, surveys etc.
- Identifying community problems and vision from bottom up in a participatory manner in the belief that the community will have greater impact on the choice of interventions;
- Identifying influential people of the community to be focal points for the possible change;
- Ensuring the flow of information from bottom up and top down;
- Developing participatory operational research agenda and disseminating the results within the community using similar approach;
- Developing information and education material with cross-cultural fertilization of ideas for each community;
- Maintaining a data base of vital statistics.

World Health Organization (WHO) aims to assist the nations in the implementation of the *Regional Strategy on Reproductive Health* for the accelerated decline in maternal and perinatal mortality. It has been adopted by its member states at the 47th session of the Regional Committee (AF/RC47/R5) held in September, 1997 by:

- Facilitating programme development, including needs assessment, priority setting, policy development, capacity building, resource mobilization, monitoring and evaluation;
- Networking and collaboration among countries research and innovation;
- Timely and effective technical support for ongoing national health sector reform programmes in an integrated manner;
- Catalyzing the establishment/ strengthening of existing coordination mechanisms among the key partners.
  (Reproductive health, Strategy for the African Region, 1998-2007)

Proper Maternity Care

Following scientific biomedical principles govern the modern maternity care:

- **Primary Level**: The primary health care which is the basic level of care offers antenatal care, care for normal delivery as well as the referral services. The normal deliveries can be undertaken at home or health care establishments. This decision is taken locally to allow for family customs, traditions and the geographical location.
- **Secondary Level**: The next tier is the secondary level. This first referral level of care is hospital-based. It must be ensured that the hospital is adequately equipped with essential lifesaving facilities so as to cater to the needs of case referrals, handle complicated pregnancies and deliveries and also to take care of puerperal complications.
- **Tertiary Level**: At this level, a very small minority who is in need of highly specialized care and others requiring intensive care are managed. At the tertiary level, services of specialist are concentrated.

It is necessary to ensure linkages between all the three tiers. The maximum care needed and provided is at the primary and first referral levels to reduce maternal mortality. The health care personnel available here are midwives, nurses including community, public health and auxiliary nurses and general duty doctors trained to perform basic obstetric functions such as operative deliveries. The midwives will be the crucial staff.

Nevertheless, WHO believes that reduction in maternal mortality rates is possible through the effective application of existing knowledge, appropriate use of technology and better and optimum management of resources. However, for the successful implementation of the relevant reforms in health and education sector, in maintaining better allocation and utilization of incomes generated and in tackling the problems of social malaise and disruption, strong political will is the prerequisite.

Barriers and Challenges

Despite these opportunities, a series of multifaceted barriers currently prohibits good sexual and reproductive health for adolescents. At the **political level**, Adolescent Sexual and Reproductive Health (ASRH) is a low priority area with restrictive laws and policies. In addition, different societal, cultural and religious factors create an unconducive environment for ASRH discussion due to deep-rooted attitude of disapproval for adolescent sexual activity. This is usually demonstrated by stigmatizing sexual health concerns, particularly STI's / HIV concerns. There is an abundance of judgmental attitudes about sexual activity, especially for those who are out of marriage and those girls and women who are sexually active. There may also be well accepted early marriage and childbearing practices in some regions, age differences between partners and societal pressure prohibiting the use of contraceptive methods. Further, conflict, migration, urbanization and lack of schooling also confound the problems leading to poor ASRH.

In terms of service-related barriers, there are poor health systems for sexual and reproductive health, family planning and maternal health, ignoring the needs of unmarried adolescents in some cases, married adolescents in others and a general lack of youth-friendly services. There is a lack of integration where counseling and family planning services do not include HIV / STI care, etc. Corruption and a lack / erratic availability of supplies and equipment may also hamper these services. Economic and physical accessibility also restricts an access to services for adolescents wherever these do exist.

On a **personal level**, the fear (of people finding out and other confidentiality issues that may result in violence), embarrassment, lack of knowledge, misinformation and myths, stigma and shame restrict the young people's care-seeking behavior (Blanc et al, 2009). Adolescents' access to information and services is influenced by a range of people, including peers, parents, family members, teachers and healthcare workers. However, some consider the attitude of health care providers as the single most important barrier to health care (International Federation of Gynecology and Obstetrics, 2011). Moreover, many adolescents are deterred by healthcare workers from using these services due to lack of confidentiality, judgmental attitudes, disrespect or not taking their needs seriously.

Opportunities and Potential Solutions

However, the opportunities for improving Adolescent Sexual and Reproductive Health (ASRH) come from myriad directions. With regard to services, an access to quality youth friendly, integrated services must be ensured, which should be provided by healthcare workers who have been trained to deal with adolescents. Sex education programs should be expanded, offering accurate, comprehensive information while building sexual behavior negotiation skills (Bearinger et al, 2007). Healthcare workers should be trained to provide accurate and balanced sex education, including information on contraception and condoms so that young people have the means to protect themselves, provided without stigma or judgment, in a context of healthy sexuality.

Healthcare workers influence the formulation of policy and ensure the provision of health care services for those in need of it. For example, healthcare workers should ensure to provide early and tailor-made prenatal services to young pregnant women so as to address their high risk pregnancy and redress the specific problems of anemia, malaria, HIV, and other STIs, as well as providing special attention during obstetric care, under the given conditions that they are most at risk of complications and death.

This area requires many other improvements, especially political and legal maneuvering. Healthcare workers can advocate for legal abortions, adequate post-abortion care services for young people where abortion is prohibited or adolescents have difficulty in accessing legal abortions, contraception provision for all who have an unmet need. Other Adolescent Sexual and Reproductive Health initiatives can also have a direct and long lasting impact on adolescent health and the health of their offsprings.

Mueller et al (2017) provided an overview and description of implementation activities of the multi-component, community-wide initiatives of the Teenage Pregnancy Prevention (TPP) Program initiated in the year 2010 by the Office of Adolescent Health (OAH) and the Centers for Disease Control and Prevention (CDCP). Community-wide initiatives have applied the Interactive Systems Framework (ISF) for dissemination and implementation through training and technical assistance on key elements of the initiative i.e. implementing evidence-based teen pregnancy prevention (TPP) interventions; improvement of quality and access to youth-friendly reproductive health services; education of TPP stakeholders; working with youth in communities most at risk of teen pregnancy and mobilizing the community participation to garner its support. With nearly 12,000 hours of training and technical assistance provided, the majority was for the selection, implementation and evaluation of a TPP program which is based on evidence. Implementation into real world of a community-wide approach to TPP is effort and time consuming. The findings of this study highlight the implementation of each of the components and shares experiences during planning and implementation phases of the initiative.

This community-wide initiative for teen pregnancy prevention was a ground-breaking effort to incorporate comprehensive approaches to a public health problem using tiered Training and Technical Assistance (TTA) based on the Interactive Systems Framework.

It was observed that implementation in a comprehensive manner is time consuming. It must be ensured that organizations have the ability to integrate practitioner-level best practices and strategies. This community-wide approach has the potential to push TPP forward and is also applicable to other public health issues. The new funding opportunity announcements issued by the OAH and the CDC in spring 2015 incorporated elements of community-wide initiatives and lessons learnt in order to better meet the needs of youth in communities and further reduce teenage pregnancy and birth rates (Mueller et al, 2017).

Despite various complex socio-cultural and economic factors contributing to maternal mortality in the developing world, some promising solutions do exist. The World Bank's involvement in the SOML (Saving One Million Lives) initiative in Nigeria is an example of a potentially effective model. This project uses a funding instrument, known as the Program-for-Results, under which the support is only distributed to local and state governments when clearly defined and measurable goals have been achieved. Under the SOML initiative, such goals include higher rates of skilled birth attendants and improved antenatal care quality at local health centres. World Bank monitors the progress towards these and other goals so as to assess whether the initiative's intended benefits are being provided to the poorest 40 percent of the population. With its emphasis on measurable outcomes, increased accountability and improved management, this program provides a useful model for other maternal health care programs around the world (World Bank, 2015).

Every day, approximately 830 women die from preventable causes related to pregnancy and childbirth and 99 percent of all maternal deaths occur in the developing countries. Severe bleeding (mostly bleeding after birth), infections (usually after birth), high blood pressure during pregnancy (pre-eclampsia and eclampsia), complications from delivery and unsafe abortions are the major complications that account for almost 75 percent of all maternal deaths. For this reason, the **Helping Mothers Survive (HMS)** suite of modules, developed by Jhpiego, has been implemented by **Project C.U.R.E.** to reduce maternal mortality so that babies will not have to survive without their mothers. The Helping Mothers Survive (HMS) suite of training programs provides health workers with skills in prevention, detection and management of the leading causes of maternal deaths. HMS Bleeding After Birth Complete training covers communication and teamwork, active third stage management of labour, early detection and basic management of PPH and advanced care skills such as shock management, uterine balloon tamponade, manual placenta removal, repair of cervical lacerations, and use of non-pneumatic anti-shock garment. For five years, through the Helping Babies Survive suite of modules developed by the American Academy of Pediatrics curriculum, Project C.U.R.E. has made a significant impact on the survival of new-borns alongside the international partners through the training of midwives, nurses and birth attendants. Its focus is on developing local Master Trainers who continue to train nurses and midwives and continue updating skills in their facilities (Say, 2014).

It is estimated that 60 to 70 per cent of infant deaths in Tanzania occur during the first hour of life. Of total deaths, about one-third is due to birth asphyxia, a condition in which the baby is not getting enough placental oxygen during the birth process. This condition can be damaging to the brain of the infant and is often fatal. Birth asphyxia is the most frequent cause of perinatal death (stillbirth or early neonatal death) in Tanzania, as per the global estimates. Additionally, this condition is less likely to be treated with fewer health resources in rural, poor and developing nations such as Tanzania. **Helping Babies Breathe (HBB)** is a low-cost, global initiative started in 2009 with the objective to reduce deaths from birth asphyxia and other respiratory complications at the time of birth. These life-saving techniques include stimulation of the infant, suction of the nose and mouth when appropriate and the use of a bag-valve-mask to improve respiration and circulate oxygen. The US Centers for Disease Control and Prevention (CDC) is supported by the CDC Foundation in monitoring closely the implementation of HBB in the Tanzanian Kigoma region. In Kigoma, HBB is implemented in partnership with Thamini Uhai, a Tanzanian non-governmental organization working to improve maternal and neonatal health. Kigoma is a low resource region with higher maternal and neonatal deaths as compared to other regions in the country. Though HBB itself is a very effective technique but key to its effectiveness is the manner in which the training is conducted (Perry, 2017).

Several alternative service approaches improve the health care system for adolescents and women by making these services more accessible, acceptable, appropriate, effective and equitable. Such alternative service approaches are particularly crucial to support healthy development for those adolescents and women who are particularly at high risk and more vulnerable to bad health or unhealthy habits and risky behaviors because of their demographic characteristics or other conditions. However, the health outcomes associated with such alternative service approaches is not supported by available evidence. Therefore, there is a need to identify areas of concern in which research could yield knowledge that would support qualitative improvement in the organization and delivery of health care services for adolescents and young women.

CONCLUSION

Compromising on the health of pregnant women will negatively influence the economy of a nation. Failure to invest in their health will increase the dependents in the coming generations and negatively influence the health of coming generations. It is therefore, imperative to focus on their health so as to ensure a healthier outcome for the coming generations. Moreover, Sustainable Development Goals provide an opportunity for focused attention to cater to the health care needs of pregnant women through strengthening of health care systems. To make progress towards universal health coverage, health sector needs to transform how the health system responds to the needs of the beneficiaries. A number of transitions in the delivery of services, workforce capacity and adequate financing is needed. Three types of interventions are required for increasing the utilization of services i.e. some changes in the health facilities, changes in the attitude of providers and the sensitization of the caregivers and the community to enable pregnant women to successfully manage their pregnancies.

REFERENCES

Alkema, L., Kantorova, V., Menozzi, C., & Biddlecom, A. (2013). National, regional and global rates and trends in contraceptive prevalence and unmet need for family planning between 1990 and 2015: A systematic and comprehensive analysis. *Lancet*, *381*(9878), 1642–1652. doi:10.1016/S0140-6736(12)62204-1 PMID:23489750

Bearinger, L. H., Sieving, R. E., Ferguson, J., & Sharma, V. (2007). Global perspectives on the sexual and reproductive health of adolescents: Patterns, prevention, and potential. *Lancet*, *369*(9568), 1220–1231. doi:10.1016/S0140-6736(07)60367-5 PMID:17416266

Blanc, A. K., Tsui, A. O., Croft, T. N., & Trevitt, J. L. (2009). Patterns and trends in adolescents' contraceptive use and discontinuation in developing countries and comparisons with adult women. *International Perspectives on Sexual and Reproductive Health*, *35*(2), 63–71. doi:10.1363/3506309 PMID:19620090

Chang, J., Elam-Evans, L. D., & Berg, C. J. (2003). Pregnancy related mortality surveillance—United States, 1991-1999. *MMWR. Surveillance Summaries, 52*, 1–8. PMID:12825542

Chen, X. K., Wen, S. W., Fleming, N., Demissie, K., Rhoads, G. G., & Walker, M. (2007). Teenage pregnancy and adverse birth outcomes: A large population based retrospective cohort study. *International Journal of Epidemiology, 36*(2), 368–373. doi:10.1093/ije/dyl284 PMID:17213208

Coco, L., Giannone, T. T., & Zarbo, G. (2014). Management of high-risk pregnancy. *Minerva Ginecologica, 66*(4), 383–389. PMID:25020057

Coyne, C.A. & D'Onofrio, B.M. (2012). Some (but not much) progress toward understanding teenage childbearing: A review of research from the past decade. *Advances in Child Development and Behaviour, 42*, 113-52.

Hall, M. H., & Bewley, S. (1999). Maternal mortality and mode of delivery. *Lancet, 354*(9180), 776. doi:10.1016/S0140-6736(05)76016-5 PMID:10475219

Harper, M. A., Byington, R. P., Espeland, M. A., Naughton, M., Meyer, R., & Lane, K. (2003). Pregnancy-related death and health care services. *Obstetrics and Gynecology, 102*, 273. PMID:12907099

Hodgkinson, S. C., Colantuoni, E., Roberts, D., Berg-Cross, L., & Belcher, H. M. (2010). Depressive symptoms and birth outcomes among pregnant teenagers. *Journal of Pediatric and Adolescent Gynecology, 23*(1), 16–22. doi:10.1016/j.jpag.2009.04.006 PMID:19679498

International Federation of Gynecology and Obstetrics. (2011). *Adolescent sexual and reproductive health (ASRH).* London: FIGO. https://www.go.org/. go-projectpublications

Korenman, S., & Fales, S. (2011). *The socioeconomic effects of teenage childbearing: A review of the recent literature.* Baruch College, City University of New York.

Lawlor, D. A., Mortensen, L., & Andersen, A. M. (2011). Mechanisms underlying the associations of maternal age with adverse perinatal outcomes: A sibling study of 264 695 Danish women and their firstborn offspring. *International Journal of Epidemiology, 40*(5), 1205–1214. doi:10.1093/ije/dyr084 PMID:21752786

Lopez, L. M., Hiller, J. E., & Grimes, D. A. (2012). Education for contraceptive use by women after childbirth. *Cochrane Database of Systematic Reviews, 8*, CD001863. PMID:22895923

Mueller, T., Tevendale, H. D., & Taleria, R. (2017). Teen pregnancy prevention: Implementation of a multicomponent, community-wide approach. *The Journal of Adolescent Health, 60*(3), S9–S17. doi:10.1016/j.jadohealth.2016.11.002 PMID:28235440

National Research Council. (2005). *Growing up global: The changing transitions to adulthood in developing countries*. The National Academies Press.

Nichols, C. (2015). *Saving Our Mothers: Enhancing Pregnancy Survival in the 21st Century*. BLOG.

Nortman, D. (1974). *Parental age as a factor in pregnancy outcome and child development. Reports on Population/Family Planning*. Population Council.

Nove, A., Matthews, Z., Neal, S. & Camacho, A.V. (2014). Maternal mortality in adolescents compared with women of other ages: evidence from 144 countries. *Lancet Global Health*. (13)70179-7. doi:10.1016/S2214-109X

Ozimek, J. A., & Kilpatrick, S. J. (2018). Maternal Mortality in the Twenty-First Century. *Obstetrics and Gynecology Clinics, 45*(2), 175–186. PMID:29747724

Perry, J. (2017). *Helping babies breathe in Tanzania*. Retrieved from https://www.cdcfoundation.org/blog/helping-babies-breathe-tanzania

Peterson, E., & Hibbard, J. U. (2018). Medical Disorders in Pregnancy. *Obstetrics and Gynecology Clinics, 45*(2), xv–xvi. PMID:29747739

Say, L., Chou, D., Gemmill, A., Tunçalp, Ö., Moller, A. B., Daniels, J. D., Gülmezoglu, A. M., Temmerman, M., & Alkema, L. (2014). Global Causes of Maternal Death: A WHO Systematic Analysis. *The Lancet. Global Health, 2*(6), e323–e333. doi:10.1016/S2214-109X(14)70227-X PMID:25103301

Sedgh, G., Finer, L. B., Bankole, A., Eilers, M. A., & Singh, S. (2015). Adolescent pregnancy, birth, and abortion rates across countries: Levels and recent trends. *The Journal of Adolescent Health, 56*(2), 223–230. doi:10.1016/j.jadohealth.2014.09.007 PMID:25620306

Singh, S. (1998). Adolescent childbearing in developing countries: A global review. *Studies in Family Planning, 29*, 117-36.

Singh, S., & Darroch, J. E. (2000). Adolescent pregnancy and childbearing: Levels and trends in developed countries. *Family Planning Perspectives*, *32*(1), 14–23. doi:10.2307/2648144 PMID:10710702

Tebeu, P. M., Fomulu, J. N., Khaddaj, S., de Bernis, L., Delvaux, T., & Rochat, C. H. (2012). Risk factors for obstetric fistula: A clinical review. *International Urogynecology Journal and Pelvic Floor Dysfunction*, *23*(4), 387–394. doi:10.100700192-011-1622-x PMID:22143450

UN Population Division. (2009). *World fertility patterns 2009.* New York: United Nations. https://www.un.org/esa/population/publications/worldfertility2009/worldfertility2009.htm

UNFPA. (2012). *By choice, not by chance: family planning, human rights and development—state of world population.* United Nations Population Fund.

UNFPA. (2013a). *Motherhood in childhood: Facing the challenge of adolescent pregnancy: The State of World Population 2013.* United Nations Population Fund.

UNFPA. (2013b). *The state of world population 2013: motherhood in childhood.* United Nations Population Fund.

World Bank. (2015). *Nigeria—Saving One Million Lives Initiative Program-for-Results (PforR) Project.* Washington, DC: World Bank Group. https://documents.worldbank.org/curated/en/2015/04/24313025/nigeria-saving-one-million-lives-initiative-program-for-results-pforr-project

World Health Organization. (2000). *Reducing Maternal Mortality: A Challenge for the 21st Century. Technical discussions.* Regional Committee for Africa Afr/Rc50/Td/1.

World Health Organization. (2011). *WHO guidelines on preventing early pregnancy and poor reproductive outcomes among adolescents in developing countries.* World Health Organization.

World Health Organization. (2013). *Accountability for maternal, newborn and child survival: The 2013 update.* World Health Organization.

World Health Organization. (2014a). *Preventing early pregnancy and poor reproductive outcomes among adolescents in developing countries.* Available at: http://www.who.int/reproductivehealth/publications/adolescence/9789241502214/en/

World Health Organization. (2014b). *Adolescent pregnancy. Fact sheet No. 364.September 2014*. Retrieved from https://www.who.int/mediacentre/factsheets/fs364/en/

World Health Organization. (2014c). Maternal, newborn, child and adolescent health. *Adolescent Pregnancy*. http://www.who.int/maternal_child_adolescent/topics/maternal/ adolescent_pregnancy/en/

World Health Organization. (2014d). *Maternal Mortality Fact Sheet*. https://www.who.int/mediacentre/factsheets/fs348/en/

World Health Organization. (2015). *MDG 5: Improve Maternal Health*. https://www.who.int/topics/millennium_development_goals/maternal_health/en/

World Health Organization, UNICEF, UNFPA, World Bank. (2010). *Trends in maternal mortality: 1990 to 2008*. World Health Organization.

Glossary

ACOG: American College of Obstetrics and Gynecology

ACTH: Adreno Cortico Tropic Hormone

ADA: American Diabetes Association

ADH: Anti Diuretic Hormone

ADHD: Attention Deficit Hyperactivity Disorder

AFE: Amniotic Fluid Embolism

AHRQ: Agency for Healthcare Research and Quality

AIDS: Auto Immune Disease Syndrome

AMTSL: Active Management of the Third Stage of Labor

APA: American Psychological Association

ART: Assisted Reproductive Technology

ASRH: Adolescent Sexual and Reproductive Health

AVP: Arginine Vasopressin

BMR: Basal Metabolic Rate

BPM: Beats Per Minute

CBG: Cortico-Steroid Binding Globulin

CDC: Centers for Disease Control

CDCP: Centers for Disease Control and Prevention

CPR: Cardiopulmonary Resuscitation

C-Section: Cesarean Section

CURE: Commission on Urgent Relief and Equipment

D&C: Dilation and Curettage

DALY's: Disability-Adjusted Life Years

DVT: Deep Vein Thrombosis

ECV: External Cephalic Version

EFA: Essential Fatty Acid

EmOC: Emergency Obstetric Care

FAO: Food and Agricultural Organization

FAQ: Frequently Asked Questions

FEV: Forced Expiratory Volume

FSH: Follicle Stimulating Hormone

G.I.Diet: Glycemic Index Diet

GBD: Global Burden of Disease

GCP: Glomerular Capillary Permeability

GDM: Gestational Diabetes Mellitus

GDP: Gross Domestic Product

GFR: Glomerular Filtration Rate

GNI: Gross National Income

HAPO: Hyperglycemia and Adverse Pregnancy Outcomes

HBB: Helping Babies Breath

HCG: human Chorionic Gonadotropin

HDI: Human Development Index

HG: Hyperemesis Gravidarum

HHS: Health and Human Services

HIV: Human Immunodeficiency Virus

HMS: Helping Mother Survive

ICDS: Integrated Child Development Services

ICMR: Indian Council of Medical Research

ICPD: International Conference on Population and Development

IDA: Iron Deficiency Anaemia

IDD: Iodine Deficiency Disorder

IPPF: International Planned Parenthood Federation

ISF: Interactive Systems Framework

IUGR: Intra Uterine Growth Retardation

IV: Intravenous

IVF: In Vitro Fertilization

LBW: Low Birth Weight

LDL: Low Density Lipoprotein

LGBT: Lesbian, Gay, Bisexual, and Transgender

LH: Luteinising Hormone

LMIC: Low Middle Income Countries

MCH: Maternal and Child Health

MDG: Millennium Development Goals

MHFW: Ministry of Health and Family Welfare

Ml/min: Millilitre/minute

Mmol/l: Micromole/litre

MMR: Maternal Mortality Rate

MMWR: Morbidity and Mortality Weekly Reports

MTP: Medical Termination of Pregnancy

MUSC: Medical University of South Carolina

NAM: National Academy of Medicine

NCHS: National Center for Health Statistics

NFHS: National Family Health Survey

NHS: National Health Service

NICE: National Institute for Clinical Excellence

NICHD: National Institute of Child Health and Human Development

NICU: Neonatal Intensive Care Unit

NIDDK: National Institute of Diabetes and Digestive and Kidney Diseases

NIN: National Institute of Nutrition

OAH: Office of Adolescent Health

OGTT: Oral Glucose Tolerance Test

ORT: Oral Rehydration Therapy

PATH: Program for Appropriate Technology in Health

PCOD: Poly Cystic Ovarian Syndrome

PE: Pulmonary Thromboembolism

PEFR: Peak Expiratory Flow Rate

pH: Negative Logrithum of Hydrogen Ion Concentration

PICC: Peripherally Inserted Central Catheter

PoA: Program of Action

PPH: Post-Partum Hemorrhage

PTSD: Post Traumatic Stress Disorder

PUL: Pregnancy of Unknown Location

RBC: Red Blood Corpuscles

RDA: Recommended Dietary Allowances

Rh-ve: Rhesus Negative

RPF: Renal Plasma Flow

SLE: Systemic Lupus Erythematosus

SOGC: Society of Obstetricians and Gynaecologists of Canada

SOML: Saving One Million Lives

SRHS: Sexual and Reproductive Health Services

SSA: Sub-Saharan Africa

STD's: Sexually Transmitted Diseases

TAA: Training and Technical Assistance

TAH: Trust for America's Health

TBA: Traditional Birth Attendant

TBG: Thyroxine Binding Globulin

TCF7LZ: Transcription Factor 7-like 2

TPP: Teen Pregnancy Prevention

TSH: Thyroid Stimulating Hormone

UK: United Kingdom

UN: United Nations

UNFPA: United Nations Family Planning Association

UNICEF: United Nations Children's Fund

USA: United States of America

USAID: United States Agency for International Development

VLBW: Very Low Birth Weight

VTE: Venous Thromboembolism

WHO: World Health Organization

Related Readings

To continue IGI Global's long-standing tradition of advancing innovation through emerging research, please find below a compiled list of recommended IGI Global book chapters and journal articles in the numerous areas related to high-risk pregnancies. These related readings will provide additional information and guidance to further enrich your knowledge and assist you with your own research.

Adcock, A., Cram, F., & Lawton, B. (2019). E Hine. In D. Akella (Ed.), *Socio-Cultural Influences on Teenage Pregnancy and Contemporary Prevention Measures* (pp. 250–272). IGI Global. doi:10.4018/978-1-5225-6108-8.ch014

Akella, D. (2019). Bringing Culture Back. In D. In Akella (Ed.), *Socio-Cultural Influences on Teenage Pregnancy and Contemporary Prevention Measures* (pp. 273–292). IGI Global. doi:10.4018/978-1-5225-6108-8.ch015

Akella, D. (2019). Situating Foucault in Teenage Pregnancy Prevention Measures. In D. Akella (Ed.), *Socio-Cultural Influences on Teenage Pregnancy and Contemporary Prevention Measures* (pp. 234–248). IGI Global. doi:10.4018/978-1-5225-6108-8.ch013

Akella, N. R. (2019). At the Mercy of Facebook. In D. Akella (Ed.), *Socio-Cultural Influences on Teenage Pregnancy and Contemporary Prevention Measures* (pp. 129–149). IGI Global. doi:10.4018/978-1-5225-6108-8.ch008

Aktan, E. (2019). Blogger Mothers as a Transmediatic Narration. In R. Yılmaz, M. N. Erdem, & F. Resuloğlu (Eds.), *Handbook of Research on Transmedia Storytelling and Narrative Strategies* (pp. 251–270). IGI Global. doi:10.4018/978-1-5225-5357-1.ch013

Al-Khasawneh, A., & Hijazi, H. (2019). Classifying Diabetes Disease Using Feedforward MLP Neural Networks. In N. Dey (Ed.), *Technological Innovations in Knowledge Management and Decision Support* (pp. 127–149). IGI Global. doi:10.4018/978-1-5225-6164-4.ch006

Bagasra, O., & Bagasra, A. (2019). Exposure to Toxic Environmental Agents in the Form of Fragrances and Development of Autism Spectrum Disorders (ASD). In P. Papadopoulou, C. Marouli, & A. Misseyanni (Eds.), *Environmental Exposures and Human Health Challenges* (pp. 52–85). IGI Global. doi:10.4018/978-1-5225-7635-8.ch003

Bata, H. (2019). Technology and Teenage Pregnancy. In D. Akella (Ed.), *Socio-Cultural Influences on Teenage Pregnancy and Contemporary Prevention Measures* (pp. 150–164). IGI Global. doi:10.4018/978-1-5225-6108-8.ch009

Beaudoin, S. (2019). The Hidden Face of Medical Intervention. In C. Albuquerque (Ed.), *Emerging Trends and Innovations in Privacy and Health Information Management* (pp. 188–211). IGI Global. doi:10.4018/978-1-5225-8470-4.ch008

Boateng, J. K. (2019). Education, Social Capital, Physical, and Psychological Access to Healthcare Among Female Migrants in Informal Settlements in Accra City, Ghana. In I. Biao (Ed.), *Learning Cities, Town Planning, and the Creation of Livelihoods* (pp. 205–232). IGI Global. doi:10.4018/978-1-5225-8134-5.ch012

Carlin, P. M. (2020). Parental Leave During Surgical Training. In M. I. Bellini & V. E. Papalois (Eds.), *Gender Equity in the Medical Profession* (pp. 16–28). IGI Global. doi:10.4018/978-1-5225-9599-1.ch002

Dandotiya, B. (2019). Health Effects of Air Pollution in Urban Environment. In A. Karmaoui (Ed.), *Climate Change and Its Impact on Ecosystem Services and Biodiversity in Arid and Semi-Arid Zones* (pp. 96–115). IGI Global. doi:10.4018/978-1-5225-7387-6.ch006

Dearden, J. C. (2019). Prediction of Human Lethality of Psychoactive Drugs From Rodent LD50 Values. *International Journal of Quantitative Structure-Property Relationships*, *4*(2), 1–27. doi:10.4018/IJQSPR.2019040101

Delgado, J. E., & Boncheva, A. I. (2018). Labor Protection in Mexico. In S. Amine (Ed.), *Employment Protection Legislation in Emerging Economies* (pp. 99–122). IGI Global. doi:10.4018/978-1-5225-4134-9.ch005

Fields, M. D. (2019). Women in American Labour Movement. *International Journal of Public and Private Perspectives on Healthcare, Culture, and the Environment*, *3*(2), 59–66. doi:10.4018/IJPPPHCE.2019070104

Golman, M., Ricks, N., Gallegos, I. D., & Weaver, J. (2019). Utilizing the Socio-Ecologic Model as a Framework for the Prevention of Teen Pregnancy. In D. Akella (Ed.), *Socio-Cultural Influences on Teenage Pregnancy and Contemporary Prevention Measures* (pp. 208–233). IGI Global. doi:10.4018/978-1-5225-6108-8.ch012

Gordon, K. C. (2020). Breaking out of the Ivory Tower. In R. F. Kronick (Ed.), *Emerging Perspectives on Community Schools and the Engaged University* (pp. 157–172). IGI Global. doi:10.4018/978-1-7998-0280-8.ch010

Halder, D. (2020). Pregnancy Vlogs and Online Victimisation of Women. In J. O. Ayodele (Ed.), *Global Perspectives on Victimization Analysis and Prevention* (pp. 40–53). IGI Global. doi:10.4018/978-1-7998-1112-1.ch003

Hamrick, J., DiGangi, E. A., Travers, J., & DiGangi, S. A. (2020). Recommendations for Implementing Comprehensive Sexuality Education for Students With Autism and Other Developmental Disabilities. In P. S. Whitby (Ed.), *Cases on Teaching Sexuality Education to Individuals With Autism* (pp. 237–253). IGI Global. doi:10.4018/978-1-7998-2987-4.ch014

Handwerk, S. E., & Handwerk, K. (2019). Teenage Pregnancy. In D. Akella (Ed.), *Socio-Cultural Influences on Teenage Pregnancy and Contemporary Prevention Measures* (pp. 1–32). IGI Global. doi:10.4018/978-1-5225-6108-8.ch001

Harries, R. L., Nicholas, R. S., & Mohan, H. M. (2020). Supporting Surgeons to Have Families. In M. I. Bellini & V. E. Papalois (Eds.), *Gender Equity in the Medical Profession* (pp. 1–15). IGI Global. doi:10.4018/978-1-5225-9599-1.ch001

Harris, K. R., & Hopper, M. T. (2019). Preventing Teen Pregnancy at Pre-Adolescence. In D. Akella (Ed.), *Socio-Cultural Influences on Teenage Pregnancy and Contemporary Prevention Measures* (pp. 166–188). IGI Global. doi:10.4018/978-1-5225-6108-8.ch010

Heisler, C. A., Stephens, E. H., Temkin, S. M., & Miller, P. (2020). Gender Inequity in the United States Surgical Workforce. In M. I. Bellini & V. E. Papalois (Eds.), *Gender Equity in the Medical Profession* (pp. 252–269). IGI Global. doi:10.4018/978-1-5225-9599-1.ch018

Heisler, E. (2017). Measuring Enclosures and Efficacy in Online Feminism. In Handbook of Research on Citizen Engagement and Public Participation in the Era of New Media (pp. 389-409). IGI Global. http://doi:10.4018/978-1-5225-1081-9.ch021

Huidu, A. (2019). The Ethics of Embrionic Stem Cells Research. In A. Sandu, A. Frunza, & E. Unguru (Eds.), *Ethics in Research Practice and Innovation* (pp. 244–263). IGI Global. doi:10.4018/978-1-5225-6310-5.ch013

Jordan, M. (2019). A Methodological Consideration and Methodological Design Suitable to Examine Teenage Pregnancy. In D. Akella (Ed.), *Socio-Cultural Influences on Teenage Pregnancy and Contemporary Prevention Measures* (pp. 33–42). IGI Global. doi:10.4018/978-1-5225-6108-8.ch002

Kim, W. J., Kim, I. K., Kim, J., & Kim, M. (2018). UX Design Guideline for Health Mobile Application to Improve Accessibility for the Visually Impaired. In S. Paiva (Ed.), *Mobile Applications and Solutions for Social Inclusion* (pp. 288–309). IGI Global. doi:10.4018/978-1-5225-5270-3.ch012

Kumar, D. (2020). Health and Well-Being Among the Jats of Western Uttar Pradesh. In S. Padmanaban & C. Subudhi (Eds.), *Psycho-Social Perspectives on Mental Health and Well-Being* (pp. 136–160). IGI Global. doi:10.4018/978-1-7998-1185-5.ch007

Kumar, S. U., Azar, A. T., Inbarani, H. H., Liyaskar, O. J., & Almustafa, K. M. (2019). Weighted Rough Set Theory for Fetal Heart Rate Classification. *International Journal of Sociotechnology and Knowledge Development*, *11*(4), 1–19. doi:10.4018/IJSKD.2019100101

Lejbkowicz, I. (2020). Web-Based Information for Patients and Providers. In R. W. McHaney, I. Reychev, J. Azuri, M. E. McHaney, & R. Moshonov (Eds.), *Impacts of Information Technology on Patient Care and Empowerment* (pp. 19–33). IGI Global. doi:10.4018/978-1-7998-0047-7.ch002

Lorraine-Lichtenstein, E. (2020). Gender Equity in Medicine in Sweden. In M. I. Bellini & V. E. Papalois (Eds.), *Gender Equity in the Medical Profession* (pp. 213–229). IGI Global. doi:10.4018/978-1-5225-9599-1.ch015

Luk, C. Y. (2019). A Human Rights-Based Approach to Teenage Pregnancy Prevention in China. In D. Akella (Ed.), *Socio-Cultural Influences on Teenage Pregnancy and Contemporary Prevention Measures* (pp. 95–116). IGI Global. doi:10.4018/978-1-5225-6108-8.ch006

Manan, A. (2020). Islamic Educational Values in Life-Cycle Rituals. In M. Huda, J. Safar, A. K. Mohamed, K. A. Jasmi, & B. Basiron (Eds.), *Global Perspectives on Teaching and Learning Paths in Islamic Education* (pp. 118–134). IGI Global. doi:10.4018/978-1-5225-8528-2.ch007

Miszczyńska, K. M. (2020). Challenges and Opportunities of the Sustainability in Healthcare. In M. Ziolo (Ed.), *Social, Economic, and Environmental Impacts Between Sustainable Financial Systems and Financial Markets* (pp. 120–149). IGI Global. doi:10.4018/978-1-7998-1033-9.ch007

Monyai, R. B., & Metsing, K. M. (2019). Understanding Teenage Pregnancy in the South African Context. In D. Akella (Ed.), *Socio-Cultural Influences on Teenage Pregnancy and Contemporary Prevention Measures* (pp. 117–128). IGI Global. doi:10.4018/978-1-5225-6108-8.ch007

Nandamuri, P. P., Jain, R. R., & Gnanamkonda, V. (2018). Corporate Supply Chains and the Challenge of Labor Standards. In U. Akkucuk (Ed.), *Handbook of Research on Supply Chain Management for Sustainable Development* (pp. 75–103). IGI Global. doi:10.4018/978-1-5225-5757-9.ch005

Oliveira, S. M. (2020). Talking About Rare Diseases. In L. V. Costa & S. Oliveira (Eds.), *Communicating Rare Diseases and Disorders in the Digital Age* (pp. 1–86). IGI Global. doi:10.4018/978-1-7998-2088-8.ch001

Olmos, S., & Nares, J. J. (2020). Applying Fault Trees to the Analysis at the Minimum Age for Sexual Consent in the Criminal Law of México. In A. Balloni & R. Sette (Eds.), *Handbook of Research on Trends and Issues in Crime Prevention, Rehabilitation, and Victim Support* (pp. 60–78). IGI Global. doi:10.4018/978-1-7998-1286-9.ch005

Olukolu, Y. R. (2017). Harmful Traditional Practices, Laws, and Reproductive Rights of Women in Nigeria. In D. Halder & K. Jaishankar (Eds.), *Therapeutic Jurisprudence and Overcoming Violence Against Women* (pp. 1–14). IGI Global. doi:10.4018/978-1-5225-2472-4.ch001

Opiyo, V. A., & Ives, Y. (2017). Relationship Literacy. In N. R. Silton (Ed.), *Family Dynamics and Romantic Relationships in a Changing Society* (pp. 168–192). IGI Global. doi:10.4018/978-1-5225-2404-5.ch009

Pande, V. S. (2020). Contribution of Men in Safe Motherhood. *International Journal of Public and Private Perspectives on Healthcare, Culture, and the Environment*, *4*(1), 27–40. doi:10.4018/IJPPPHCE.2020010103

Paraskou, A., & George, B. (2018). *Theoretical Framework*. IGI Global. doi:10.4018/978-1-5225-2694-0.ch002

Ramakrishnan, S. & Jayaraman, A. (2019). Pesticide Contaminated Drinking Water and Health Effects on Pregnant Women and Children. In Handbook of Research on the Adverse Effects of Pesticide Pollution in Aquatic Ecosystems (pp. 123-136). IGI Global. http://doi:10.4018/978-1-5225-6111-8.ch007

Ramulumo, M. R. (2019). Causes and Factors Responsible for Teenage Pregnancy. In D. Akella (Ed.), *Socio-Cultural Influences on Teenage Pregnancy and Contemporary Prevention Measures* (pp. 44–63). IGI Global. doi:10.4018/978-1-5225-6108-8.ch003

Rausch, M. A., & Wikoff, H. D. (2020). Case Study for Counseling Same Sex Couples Through the Fertility Process. In B. C. King & T. A. Stewart (Eds.), *Cases on Cross-Cultural Counseling Strategies* (pp. 66–88). IGI Global. doi:10.4018/978-1-7998-0022-4.ch004

Rouhani, S., & Maryam MirSharif. (2018). Data Mining Approach for the Early Risk Assessment of Gestational Diabetes Mellitus. *International Journal of Knowledge Discovery in Bioinformatics*, *8*(1), 1–11. doi:10.4018/IJKDB.2018010101

Rua, M., Leal, R. M., & Costa, N. (2019). Multimodal Narratives in Nursing Education. In J. B. Lopes, M. C. Viegas, & J. A. Pinto (Eds.), *Multimodal Narratives in Research and Teaching Practices* (pp. 356–375). IGI Global. doi:10.4018/978-1-5225-8570-1.ch018

Saeed, N., Khan, S. K., Raheed, H. M., & Hussain, M. Z. (2018). Empirical Analysis of Socio-economic Factors Effecting Nutritional Status of Children (1-5) of Age. *International Journal of Civic Engagement and Social Change*, *5*(4), 1–18. doi:10.4018/IJCESC.2018100101

Saeed, N., Rehman, T. U., & Usmani, M. A. (2018). Impact of Socioeconomic Factors on the Nutritional Status of Elementary School's Children in Rural Areas of Karachi (Pakistan). *International Journal of Civic Engagement and Social Change*, *5*(2), 36–47. doi:10.4018/IJCESC.2018040102

Sakr, M. (2020). *Clinical Course*. IGI Global. doi:10.4018/978-1-5225-9655-4.ch008

Sakr, M. (2020). *Dietary Management*. IGI Global. doi:10.4018/978-1-5225-9655-4.ch015

Sakr, M. (2020). *Etiology and Risk Factors*. IGI Global. doi:10.4018/978-1-5225-9655-4.ch005

Sarigiannis, D. A. (2019). The Exposome Paradigm in Environmental Health. In P. Papadopoulou, C. Marouli, & A. Misseyanni (Eds.), *Environmental Exposures and Human Health Challenges* (pp. 1–29). IGI Global. doi:10.4018/978-1-5225-7635-8.ch001

Sarigiannis, D. A., Gotti, A. C., & Karakitsios, S. P. (2019). The Waste-Energy-Health Nexus. In P. Papadopoulou, C. Marouli, & A. Misseyanni (Eds.), *Environmental Exposures and Human Health Challenges* (pp. 297–342). IGI Global. doi:10.4018/978-1-5225-7635-8.ch014

Sarper, N. (2020). Health Literacy From a Pediatrician's Perspective. In N. O. Taskiran (Ed.), *Handbook of Research on Multidisciplinary Approaches to Literacy in the Digital Age* (pp. 308–330). IGI Global. doi:10.4018/978-1-7998-1534-1.ch015

Shema, C. R. (2019). Psychosocial and Cultural Contributing Factors of Teen Pregnancy in North America. In D. Akella (Ed.), *Socio-Cultural Influences on Teenage Pregnancy and Contemporary Prevention Measures* (pp. 64–76). IGI Global. doi:10.4018/978-1-5225-6108-8.ch004

Sikulibo, J. (2019). *The Crimes of Sexual Violence in the Jurisprudence of International Criminal Tribunals*. IGI Global. doi:10.4018/978-1-5225-8194-9.ch002

Srinivasan, R. (2018). Women, Armed Conflicts, and Violence. In R. C. Das (Ed.), *Handbook of Research on Military Expenditure on Economic and Political Resources* (pp. 472–494). IGI Global. doi:10.4018/978-1-5225-4778-5.ch024

Srivastava, K. (2019). Autism and Diet. In S. K. Gupta, S. Venkatesan, S. Goswami, & R. Kumar (Eds.), *Emerging Trends in the Diagnosis and Intervention of Neurodevelopmental Disorders* (pp. 194–210). IGI Global. doi:10.4018/978-1-5225-7004-2.ch010

Sucharith, P., Suprith, K. P., Kasturi, U., & Ajina, A. (2020). Applications of Fuzzy Expert Systems in Farming. In A. Kumar & M. Kalpana (Eds.), *Fuzzy Expert Systems and Applications in Agricultural Diagnosis* (pp. 50–70). IGI Global. doi:10.4018/978-1-5225-9175-7.ch004

Tadepalli, S. K., & Lakshmi, P. (2019). Application of Machine Learning and Artificial Intelligence Techniques for IVF Analysis and Prediction. *International Journal of Big Data and Analytics in Healthcare*, *4*(2), 21–33. doi:10.4018/IJBDAH.2019070102

Taiwo, T. N., & Olusola, O. O. (2018). A Review of Theoretical, Conceptual, and Methodological Issues in Public Health Communication. In A. Salawu & T. O. Owolabi (Eds.), *Exploring Journalism Practice and Perception in Developing Countries* (pp. 194–216). IGI Global. doi:10.4018/978-1-5225-3376-4.ch010

Tilaoui, M., Zyad, A., Chatoui, H., & Rakkaa, T. (2019). Childhood Leukemia and Environmental Risk Factors. In K. Kahime, M. El Hidan, O. El Hiba, D. Sereno, & L. Bounoua (Eds.), *Handbook of Research on Global Environmental Changes and Human Health* (pp. 193–214). IGI Global. doi:10.4018/978-1-5225-7775-1.ch010

Tiwari, M., Agrawal, D. S., & Mitra, S. (2017). Abnormal Uterine Bleeding (AUB) and Thyroid Function in Chhattisgarh. *International Journal of User-Driven Healthcare*, *7*(2), 29–41. doi:10.4018/IJUDH.2017070103

Tshishonga, N. S. (2019). Youth Participation and Representation in Community Governance at Cato Manor Township, Durban. In J. Kurebwa & O. Dodo (Eds.), *Participation of Young People in Governance Processes in Africa* (pp. 268–295). IGI Global. doi:10.4018/978-1-5225-9388-1.ch013

Uddin, M. N., Rahman, M. M., & Khatun, M. M. (2019). Illness Profile of a Disaster Prone Bangladeshi Village. In Q. R. Yasser (Ed.), *Handbook of Research on Rural Sociology and Community Mobilization for Sustainable Growth* (pp. 146–163). IGI Global. doi:10.4018/978-1-5225-7158-2.ch009

Vidourek, R. A., & King, K. A. (2019). Preventing Teen Pregnancy Among Minority Populations. In D. Akella (Ed.), *Socio-Cultural Influences on Teenage Pregnancy and Contemporary Prevention Measures* (pp. 189–207). IGI Global. doi:10.4018/978-1-5225-6108-8.ch011

Visser, K. (2020). Addressing the Psychosexual Development of Teenagers on the Autism Spectrum Using the Tackling Teenage Training Program. In P. S. Whitby (Ed.), *Cases on Teaching Sexuality Education to Individuals With Autism* (pp. 115–127). IGI Global. doi:10.4018/978-1-7998-2987-4.ch007

Wamalwa, A. N. (2019). Sustainable Development Goals. In A. Antonaras & P. Dekoulou (Eds.), *Cases on Corporate Social Responsibility and Contemporary Issues in Organizations* (pp. 166–182). IGI Global. doi:10.4018/978-1-5225-7715-7.ch010

Weiss-Randall, D. (2018). *Identifying and Mapping Vulnerable Populations*. IGI Global. doi:10.4018/978-1-5225-3414-3.ch003

Yildirim, F., Abukan, B., & Oztas, D. (2019). From Early Marriage to Adolescent Pregnancy in Turkey. In D. Akella (Ed.), *Socio-Cultural Influences on Teenage Pregnancy and Contemporary Prevention Measures* (pp. 77–94). IGI Global. doi:10.4018/978-1-5225-6108-8.ch005

About the Author

Sapna Nanda is a Principal in Government College of Yoga Education and Health affiliated to Panjab University, Chandigarh in India. She is Associate Professor and M.Sc. (Foods & Nutrition), M.Ed., Ph.D. and has undergone a Certificate Course in Yoga. She possesses 34 years of teaching experience at various levels i.e. Secondary, Senior Secondary and Teacher Education. She has been supervising 6 Ph.D. scholars and guided 40 dissertations at Master's Level in the areas of Nutrition, Health and Education. She has authored a research insight on *Psycho-Socio-Physical Dimensions of Adolescent Health Management: Emerging Research and Opportunities* published by IGI Global Publications of United States of America, co-authored as supervisor a book on *Intervention Strategies for ADHD* which has been published by Lambert Academic Publishing, besides three books on *Education in Contemporary India* and *Gender, School and Society* by Twentyfirst Century Publications of India as well as four edited books on *Human Rights, Quality Concerns in Teacher Education, New Education Policy: Initiatives and Implication and Curriculum Reforms in Teacher Educations. She is Chief Editor of e Journal "The Yogic Insight"*, Chief Editor of College Magazine *Kalash-The Essence of Yoga and Half Yearly Newsletter- Yog Vrittant.* Her quite a number of papers have been published in the national journals of repute and has also presented a number of papers in the National and International Conferences. Besides, a number of National Seminars/ Conferences/ Workshops/ Sponsored Projects have been organized. Her extension activities include giving lectures to NSS volunteers, anganwadi workers and supervisors of ICDS scheme, parents and community workers in the arena of Nutrition, Health, Hygiene, Yoga, Maternal, Child and Adolescent Health Care. She has been anchoring radio and television programmes on Nutrition and Health on local radio and television channels, news-reading on local television channels, Panelist of 'Swacch Bharat Abhiyaan' and 'Beti Parao-Beti Bachao' Series on Chandigarh Doordarshan in India. She is an Executive Member of Indian Dietetic Association, Chandigarh Chapter as well as the Co-editor of half yearly newsletter, Nutrition News "n" Views published by Chandigarh Chapter of Indian Dietetic Association. She is Joint Secretary of Chandigarh Softball Association. Her other professional affiliations include an added member of Faculty of Education, Panjab University, Member of Board of Studies in Health Family Welfare and Population Education, Member of Board of Studies in the Faculty of Education, Panjab University, Chandigarh and Member, Board of Studies in the Faculty of Education, Chandigarh University, Punjab, India.

Index

N

O

P

R

S

U

Y

www.ingramcontent.com/pod-product-compliance
Lightning Source LLC
LaVergne TN
LVHW081519300926
849161LV00006B/1229